Study skills and coping strategies:
A manual for international healthcare students

S Ford-Sumner

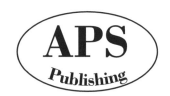

APS Publishing
The Old School, Tollard Royal, Salisbury, Wiltshire, SP5 5PW
www.apspublishing.co.uk

British Library Cataloguing in Publication Data
A catalogue record for this book is available from the British Library.

© APS Publishing 2005
ISBN 1 9038773 4 2

Printed in the United Kingdom by Cromwell Press, Trowbridge, Wiltshire

Contents

Foreword

International recruitment is currently an important element in a range of initiatives undertaken to build the NHS workforce. However, the international mobility of healthcare professionals is a well-established practice that has been going on for many years. International healthcare professionals have brought a new and valuable dimension that has enabled the transfer of experience and theory of ideas.

International mobility has also brought benefit to the individuals concerned in terms of enriching experience, skills enhancement, career opportunities and a chance to increase their quality of life. These factors help towards continuous improvements to the standards of care for patients. Their home economy can benefit when and if an individual returns home with new skills and experience.

More recent times have seen an increasingly large-scale, targeted international recruitment. One in four qualified nurses working here in London obtained their original qualifications overseas. During the year 2004–2005, over 300 qualified nurses from overseas were recruited by Trusts in East London alone. With the increasing shortfall of UK educated nurses and midwives, these numbers will only increase. The majority of these overseas-qualified nurses are educated at certificate level. Trusts and the Strategic Health Authorities have already identified the need to provide these nurses and midwives with continuing professional development (CPD) to ensure they are not disadvantaged in their career progression. Activity to support these individuals and groups here at St Bartholomew School of Nursing and Midwifery, City University include:

- The provision of a flexibly delivered supervised practice programme to meet the needs of the NHS and private sector
- Working closely with local agencies on pre supervised practice programmes
- The development of supervised practice plus programme for experienced nurses and midwives from overseas
- Co-operating with refugee nurses task groups offering counselling and education opportunities where appropriate for refugee nurses and midwives
- Providing bridging courses for overseas trained nurses who do not meet Nursing and Midwifery Council (NMC) requirements for supervised practice
- Continue to provide opportunities for overseas nurses to complete their level 2 studies.

The growth of pre-registration students from the ethnic minorities within the School also probably reflects our geographic position in the City and East London. The School's annual report for 2003 clearly shows that we recruit heavily from the black African populations and that recruitment from the local Asian populations is not in proportion to these groups' representation within the local population. Recruitment from ethnic groups of the Asian subcontinent is a recognised national issue and our local campaigns have led to significant increases in the number of applicants from these groups.

Sue Ford-Sumner, the author of this book, is currently a lecturer within the School and is therefore well placed to write a book of this nature. The book is for students of healthcare who have come to the UK from overseas to work or to study, or both; or students from overseas who have lived in the UK for a while, prior to commencing a programme of study. This book could also be of general interest to all healthcare students wishing to learn more about culture and communication, or for those who need support in relation to study skills. Teachers or mentors working with healthcare students from overseas may find this text of use when providing support for their students.

One of the book's major strengths is that throughout the experiences and views of real people who are from a variety of ethnic and professional or educational backgrounds are described. The experiences of real people help to 'bring alive' the discussion and in some instances, describe how people have adopted certain coping strategies and/or developed study skills. They also serve to highlight some of the issues encountered by international health students.

Given the context described above I cannot think of a more opportune time for a book of this nature.

Professor Sally Glen
Dean: St Bartholomew School of Nursing and Midwifery
City University

February 2005

Introduction

This chapter covers the following:

- Who could benefit from this book
- How to use this book
- The importance of communication
- English for specific purposes.

Who could benefit from this book?

You could benefit from this book if you are a student of healthcare who has come to the UK from overseas to work or to study, or both; or, you may be a student from overseas who has lived in the UK for a while, prior to commencing a programme of study. You may be a pre-registration student nurse, an adaptation nurse, you may be undertaking a health-related module as part of an undergraduate degree programme (for example the Open University degree pathway, leading to a BSc in Health and Social Care), an access course, or a course allied to healthcare. You may be a health care assistant undertaking a National Vocational Qualification (NVQ) programme.

This book could also be of general interest to all healthcare students wishing to learn more about culture and communication, or for those who need support in relation to study skills.

If you are a teacher or mentor working with healthcare students from overseas, you may find this text of use to support you in this role.

How to use this book

All chapters contain background information and a summary. Most chapters refer to the experiences and views of international healthcare students. There are activities at the end of each chapter.

You are advised, first of all, to read the background information referring to the summary in case of any difficulty. You may then like to attempt the activities. Teachers or mentors may find the activities helpful to use with students, either on an individual or group basis.

Background information

The purpose of this is to introduce you to information intended to help you to either improve your study skills, or develop coping strategies that may help you in relation to cultural adaptation. Some of this information might not be new to you, and could therefore act as revision. At the end of each section is a summary. If you have any difficulty in understanding any of the text, then this may help you.

Furthermore, there is a comprehensive glossary of the terms used throughout at the end of this book. You can refer to this if you are unsure about any of the terminology. The purpose of the glossary is to maximise the opportunity for you to make the best use of this book.

The experiences of international healthcare students

Throughout this book, the experiences and views of real people who are from a variety of ethnic and professional or educational backgrounds are described. The identities and details of all those featured have been changed, in order to ensure confidentiality and anonymity. The people represented have all given their consent. The experiences of real people help to 'bring alive' the discussion and in some instances, describe how people like you have adopted certain coping strategies and/or developed study skills. They also serve to highlight some of the issues encountered by international healthcare students.

Activities

The activities aim to help you to learn through reflection and to develop study skills and coping strategies. Many of the activities do not have 'right' or 'wrong' answers, but where appropriate, answers can be found at the back of the book in the Answers section. You should read through the background information then use the activities to make your learning more meaningful.

'I hear and I forget, I see and I remember, I do and I understand.'
Confucius

This ancient quote reflects the belief that we learn most effectively by doing—hence the importance of the activities.

Another important aspect of the activities is *reflection*. Reflection is a valuable tool to help you to think about experiences, and to learn from them. It is a tool that can be applied to both your professional and your personal life, helping you to make both more effective, productive, enjoyable and worthwhile.

One reflective tool that can be used is *critical incident analysis.* Critical incident analysis can help you to learn from your experience in a safe and structured way. Here is one example of how it has been used:

> Student nurses used critical incident analysis within the 'safe' environment of the classroom, with the guidance of an experienced facilitator. They were able to analyse incidents that had occurred during their clinical placements, in order to enhance their learning.

Many people have written about reflection. Schön (1983) compared the following:

- Knowing-in-action
- Reflection-in-action
- Reflection-on-action.

Each relates to a different way of working or functioning in some way.

Knowing-in-action

This refers to working or functioning in a way that is almost automatic, that is based on what the individual knows already, and does not involve any depth of thinking. In relation to practice it is less likely to lead to improvement, as the practitioner does not question what they do. It is however indicative of a level of knowledge and expertise.

Reflection-in-action

Reflection occurs during an event—the individual has a heightened awareness of what they are doing, as they are doing it.

Reflection-on-action

Reflection occurs after an event. This is the type of reflection that you will be asked to do within some of the activities.

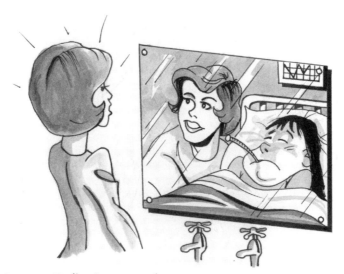

Figure Intro. 1: Reflection-on-action

You might question the purpose and value of the activities, believing that the learning required for adaptation will happen as a natural process. Of course this is true, but this type of learning is unstructured and dependent on chance. By carrying out more structured activities, you will increase the likelihood of meaningful reflection. By writing down your findings and plans, you can more objectively see what you have learned, what further areas there are for growth and development and which strategies can be used to achieve your goals.

The importance of communication

Communication is an integral part of most, if not all, activities related to healthcare. We communicate in different ways: by speaking, by writing and by using non-verbal communication, such as eye contact and gestures. Our speech is made up of recognisable words and some sounds, such as 'um' and 'err'. We use different tones of voice, in order to maintain the interest of the listener, or to emphasise a point. Increasingly, technology, in the form of mobile phones and email for example, is used to convey the spoken or the written word. Chapter 2 looks at communication types in more detail.

The following are examples of situations that involve communication:

• Carrying out an admissions interview with a patient/client

• Chatting to a patient's relative

• Discussing your progress with your mentor

• Writing an assignment

• Handing over to a colleague

• Contributing to a class discussion

• Updating a care plan

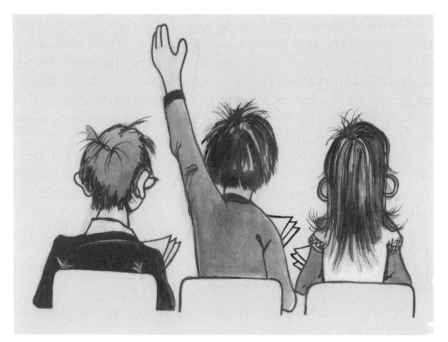

Figure Intro. 2: Contributing to a class discussion

Communication difficulties arise not only because of language problems but also because of cultural differences, which may be reflected in the colloquial and idiomatic use of language. Chapter 1 looks at the relationship between culture and communication. Chapter 2 contains information about idiomatic and colloquial language, with an emphasis on the type of language you may encounter as a healthcare student.

English for specific purposes

Other study skills texts aimed at students from overseas are generic; they are aimed at a more broad-based readership. English for Specific Purposes (ESP) is an approach derived from English as a Foreign Language (EFL) teaching. ESP programmes focus on developing communicative competence in a specific field (Hortas, accessed 2003) which in this instance is healthcare. ESP students are usually adults, and they are likely to possess an existing level of competence (Dudley-Evans, 1997). These criteria apply to those students for whom this book is intended.

This book aims to meet the specific needs of students from overseas undertaking healthcare courses by focusing primarily on the communication issues that are associated with the practice and culture of healthcare. It also recognises, however, that work or study exists within a cultural context, and that adaptation to the wider cultural context should be addressed.

Gatehouse (2001) agrees with this in that ESP programmes should address the needs of students in three areas:

- The language used within the relevant occupation (in this case, healthcare)

- The skills needed to adapt to the wider cultural context

- The skills needed to communicate on an informal basis, such as chatting to colleagues at break times.

Campbell (2001) believes that overseas nurses are most concerned with being able to communicate with patients, relatives and other nurses. He considers that the theoretical framework of ESP addresses the important language and cultural elements of these interactions.

Summary

- All international healthcare students could benefit from this book, whichever course of study they are undertaking. Some other students may find the sections on study skills helpful, and may also learn more about communication and cultural issues. Teachers and mentors could find this book a useful tool in supporting international healthcare students.

- Each chapter contains background information, including reference to the experiences of international healthcare students, a summary and activities; the summary will help to simplify information. The glossary at the back of this book should clarify any terms that you do not understand. The activities will help students to reflect and learn and are based on the premise that the most effective learning results from doing. The importance of reflection as a valuable learning tool is emphasised.

- The experiences of international healthcare students are based on real people who have consented to have their experiences adapted for this book. All contributors are international healthcare students from a variety of ethnic, professional and educational backgrounds.

- The importance of communication as an integral part of so many of our daily activities is highlighted.

- International healthcare students have specific needs in relation to cultural adaptation and communication associated with the culture and practice of healthcare. This book is informed by the principles of English for Specific Purposes (ESP) teaching which focuses on developing communicative competence in a specific field, in this case healthcare.

Chapter 1

Culture and communication

What is Culture?

'Culture' is a difficult concept to define precisely. A group of student nurses were asked the question: 'What does culture mean to you?' Their responses included:

- Values
- Beliefs
- Behaviour
- Clothing
- Religion
- Ethnicity
- Food
- Music
- Customs
- Traditions

If we look at this list, we can place these responses into two categories:

1. Those items that can be observed. These are the *symbolic* parts of a culture, for example, the type of clothing worn by a group of people;

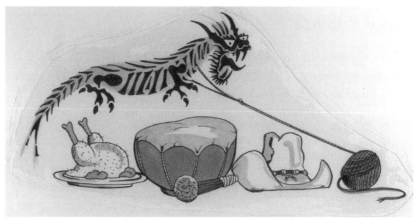

Figure 1.1a: Levels of Culture : Symbols of culture

2. Those items that cannot be observed. These include values and beliefs.

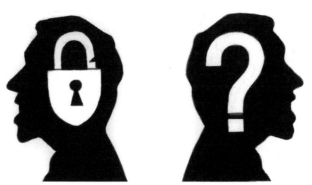

Figure 1.1b: Levels of culture: Values and beliefs cannot be observed

Often, we tend to associate 'culture' with different countries, as a concept that is applied in the wider sense. This is a *macroscopic* view of culture. Culture can also be applied to 'smaller' situations, for example to an organisation, or even a department within an organisation. This is a *microscopic* view of culture. For example, a clinical area such as a hospital ward can be said to have its own culture. Your coping strategies will include recognising aspects of the prevailing culture and devising your own 'cultural map'.

In keeping with the definitions above, within a hospital ward environment, there will be some aspects of culture that will be more obvious than others. For example:

- the routine

- ways in which people address each other

- items posted on notice boards.

These are all aspects that symbolise the prevailing culture. Your cultural map could be referred to as a representation of 'the way that things are done around here'.

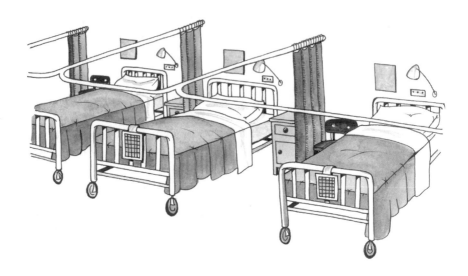

Figure 1.2: The Hospital Ward

Culture shock

In the same way that culture can be applied to different situations, so can culture shock. Culture shock refers to the sense of disorientation you may feel, having entered a different culture to the one you have been used to for a long time. You may not feel this immediately, as, initially, the novelty of a different situation may be exciting. Once the novelty wears off, you face the challenge of adapting to a new culture, which may be associated with a new country, or with a new working environment.

Many of us have encountered a degree of culture shock at some stage of our lives. Symptoms vary between individuals, but you may experience some or all of the following, depending upon the situation:

- Homesickness
- Sadness or depression
- A sense of detachment from the situation you find yourself in
- Tiredness
  - This may make it difficult for you to concentrate
- A sense of alienation, of not 'fitting in'
  - This could lead you to feel defensive.

A group of Adaptation nurses, who had recently arrived from the Philippines, were asked to identify the differences that were most obvious to them as a result of moving to the UK:

- The environment, particularly the weather
- Language differences, especially in relation to accents and pro-nunciation
- Food
- Transport.

Another group of Adaptation nurses, made up of a diversity of ethnic origin, added to this list:

- The way that people dress
- Excessive freedom
- Way of life
- 'People are more reserved'.

Yet another group made further observations:

- Currency (money) is different
- Patterns of childcare—this observation was made by an African nurse who commented that in her country, childcare is shared by the community.

Some pre-registration student nurses were also asked about the main differences they noticed when they came to the UK. Their responses included:

- More rubbish in the streets
- England not being as beautiful as expected
- Overcrowding
- The underground train system
- Increased cultural diversity.

They also agreed with many of the observations made by the Adaptation nurses.

The cultural map referred to later could be one strategy for dealing with culture shock. Other strategies include:

- Being good to yourself: taking adequate rest, eating well, exercising, treating yourself to small rewards, such as a book or favourite food
- Seeking support from others in a similar situation
- Thinking positively, trying to see this change as a challenge that you are able to face up to
- Discussing your feelings with appropriate others within your professional/educational situation. Very quickly, you will recognise those who are approachable and sympathetic,

although you should also remember that there are people whose job it is to support you in different ways. These may include:

- Your allocated mentor
- Another qualified person within your clinical placement area
- Your personal tutor
- A counsellor (counselling services are invariably provided by educational establishments providing healthcare programmes).

The group of nurses from the Philippines were asked to talk about the ways in which they had coped with their culture shock. They identified the following strategies:

- By socialising with others in the same situation
- By going out and exploring their new environment, aiming to become more orientated
- By maintaining contact with family and friends in their home country
- By keeping busy.

Again, this list was added to by the mixed-origin group:

- By being a good listener
- By making new friends
- By expressing emotion
- Shopping
- By seeking comfort from their faith

- By visiting the library.

The contribution by the groups of pre-registration student nurses, in addition to some of the above strategies, included the following:

- By some preparation before coming to a different country
- By being open to adaptation, and eager to adapt
- By receiving advice from friends and family already living in this country about certain behaviour
- By doing voluntary work prior to becoming a student nurse
- By working as a healthcare assistant prior to becoming a student nurse
- By making an effort to mix with people from a variety of backgrounds
- By using resources such as the immigration department and voluntary organisations
- By being determined to accomplish one's goals
- Support from one's partner.

Interestingly, the subject of food was discussed at some length. It was generally agreed that the groups found it difficult to locate the exact ingredients they required to make the type of meals they were accustomed to. Familiar food, it appears, can be very comforting and is one of the things that people miss most when living in a different country. Eating can also be a social event that involves sharing and conversing with others. This can therefore be integrated with socialisation, one of the identified strategies for coping with culture shock.

It is important to recognise that not all coping strategies are as positively helpful as others. For example, when people feel stressed, they cope in different ways. Some people adopt more positive strategies, such as taking exercise, using relaxation techniques or talking to others. Others adopt more negative coping strategies, such as smoking, drinking or eating too much, or by channelling their stress into aggressive behaviour.

Likewise, some people may adopt less positive strategies when trying to cope with cultural change. Most of the international students I have spoken to have expressed very positive attitudes towards cultural adaptation and, in doing so, have adopted positive coping strategies such as those previously listed. The most negative response expressed was 'keeping to myself'; a sort of avoidance tactic, minimising contact and integration with one's new environment. Obviously, each individual will respond and cope differently, but it may be helpful to take stock of how you are coping, perhaps by discussing with others.

Activity 3 on page 21 draws on this section to help you to develop strategies to adapt to a new culture more comfortably.

Cultural differences and communication issues

Part of the driving force for producing this book is the recognition that communication is not just about spoken language; it is also closely related to culture. What this means is that cultural differences may affect the ways that individuals send and receive messages.

Communication is essentially about transmitting and receiving messages. It is generally, although not always, a two-way process. Communication may be synchronous or asynchronous. Examples of synchronous communication include:

- Conversing with somebody face to face

- Talking to somebody on the telephone.

Examples of asynchronous communication include:

- Sending an email
- Opening an email
- Leaving a message on a voicemail service
- Picking up a voice message
- Sending a letter
- Reading a letter

From these examples, you can see that communication involves transmission and receipt of messages, both with and without delay between the two. Both types are susceptible to cultural influences. For example, an important element of face-to-face communication is non-verbal communication (NVC). Types of NVC include:

- Eye contact
- Facial expression
- Gesture
- Proximity/distance/space
- Touch
- Posture
- Appearance.

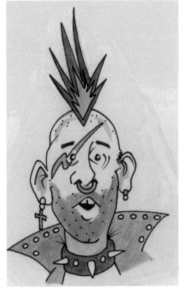

Figure 1.4: Appearance is about making a statement

There are cultural differences in NVC. For example, some African students have reported that within their cultures it is considered disrespectful to look an elder or authority figure in the eye. They go on to describe how since coming to the UK, they have learned that maintaining eye contact demonstrates interest and respect to somebody within this culture.

Some Adaptation nurses from India reported that when they first came to the UK, they noticed how the way that they nodded their heads tended to be misinterpreted. When questioned further about this, they thought that it was because instead of giving a definite 'yes' up and down head nod, they tend to move their heads in different directions, which can appear to have an ambiguous meaning.

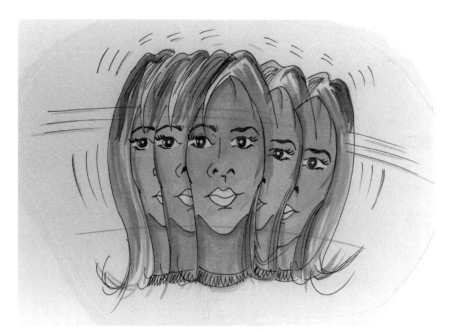

Figure 1.5: Head movements can have different meanings

So it is possible that cultural differences could unintentionally lead to misunderstandings.

At the end of this chapter are some activities that could help you to recognise situations within which misunderstandings have occurred. By reflecting on these, you can learn from them and develop strategies for coping with similar situations in the future.

Cultural issues and studying

Chapter 4 addresses issues that may arise in relation to cultural differences and studying.

Cultural issues and the workplace

If you have worked in another country, you will notice differences within the workplace, as well as those that you have observed generally. Of course, the observations that you make in the workplace will also reflect the characteristics of the wider cultural context.

Adaptation nurses have worked as qualified nurses in another country before coming to the UK and are therefore particularly likely to observe differences in work-based practices. Two groups of Adaptation nurses identified the following differences:

- The type of language used, including some medical terminology
- Some routines, for example relating to bed making and mealtimes
- Other 'rituals' such as doctors' rounds and 'lights out'
- The ways that meetings are conducted
- Referral systems
- Some practices, policies and procedures

- The type of food served to patients
- Increased reference to evidence-based practice
- A different type of involvement with relatives—more formal
- The types of clothing and fabrics used for patients
- Doctors not being as friendly, and not knowing patients' names.

It is these types of differences that make it compulsory for nurses who have trained overseas to undertake a programme of supervised practice and induction, so that they can learn more about the healthcare system in the UK, and about the policies, practices, procedures and philosophies of care with which they might be unfamiliar (NMC, 2002).

The same groups were asked to comment more specifically about the communication issues that they had experienced within their workplace in the UK. They identified the following:

- The type of language used, including some medical terminology
- Different accents
- Different sense of humour
- People speaking quickly
- The use of euphemisms. See Chapter 2 for information on this subject. An example of a practice-related euphemism identified by this group was 'not for the team', meaning that an individual is not for resuscitation
- Some staff cannot be bothered to take time to communicate with people from overseas, not making allowances for them

- Some problems understanding all of the handover,;the passing of information between shifts (this was identified by several respondents)

- The use of abbreviations. It is possible that some of these are used for the same reason as euphemisms—to disguise unpleasantness for the sake of patients. An example is 'TLC', standing for 'Tender Loving Care', a term used to denote the care that should be given to a terminally ill patient.

The activities at the end of this chapter are designed to help you to learn more about the differences you encounter within the workplace that relate to the language, culture and practice of healthcare.

Cultural maps

A cultural map is a picture that you build up of a given situation (for example a hospital ward) which describes 'the way that things are done around here'. It should help you to recognise and understand practices, and ultimately to settle in and feel part of a team. The use of cultural maps for international healthcare students has been adapted from the work of Arakelian *et al* (2003). The use of cultural maps is quite flexible and adaptable to different situations, both inside and outside of work. They could constantly change and grow as you add new experiences, and the overall picture becomes clearer.

It is important to recognise that not all cultural practices within a clinical setting are ideal; some things that you see, you may not agree with; you may feel that 'the way that things are done' does not fit comfortably with the way that you have been taught. Adaptation to a new situation should not just be about conforming, especially if this means conforming to bad practice. You should not be afraid to challenge bad practice in an appropriate way. As a student or new member of staff, you may find this difficult to do.

Furthermore, being assertive may not sit comfortably with your cultural background. For these reasons, this book includes a chapter on communication and assertiveness, in which you are shown a structured way to communicate more assertively.

Summary

- 'Culture' is made up of different components: those that are visible such as the clothes that people wear, and those that are less obvious such as values. A culture can refer to a country, a region within a country, an organisation, or a unit within an organisation, such as a hospital ward. In other words 'culture' exists at different levels.

- 'Culture shock' refers to the way that you might feel when moving to a new country or even after a significant life-change, such as starting a new job. After an initial 'honeymoon' period, you may feel disorientated and easily tired. You can adopt strategies that should help make the adaptation period easier to live through, such as looking after your physical health and seeking support from others.

- Cultural differences may affect communication. Different expectations about behaviour could lead to misunderstandings, for example in relation to some aspects of non-verbal communication, such as eye contact.

- It is possible that cultural differences may lead to difficulties in studying within a culture that is unlike the one you are accustomed to. You should always ask for clarification if anything is not clear. We have a growing number of international students from all disciplines coming to study in the UK and we need to be mindful of any problems they may experience in relation to culturally-specific teaching activities or materials.

- International healthcare students are likely to encounter differences within the workplace; these reflect the wider cultural context and may be observed as communication and practice issues.

Activities

Activity I

Devising a Cultural Map

In order to devise a cultural map, it is a good idea to carry around a small notebook and pencil at all times. When you get the opportunity, jot down notes of anything you see or hear that you find unfamiliar. This may include something that someone has said, or a practice or procedure that is unfamiliar to you. Later on, you should revise your notes and write them more neatly in a journal, including your thoughts and feelings about each item. You should then decide on a plan of action for each item. For example, someone might have used an idiomatic phrase that you do not understand (see Chapter 2). You might have asked the person immediately for clarification, in which case their response may be of interest—were they helpful or, perhaps, surprised? Did you explain that you did not understand because you are from overseas? If you did not ask for clarification, consider how you could find out more about the unfamiliar phrase. It could be that you ask your mentor, or another trusted colleague or friend. You might consult a glossary of idiomatic phrases, or the Internet. You should find out if the phrase is in frequent use, in which case you will be more likely to hear it again.

Try to do some work on your cultural map for one day. Let us imagine that you are working in a hospital ward. Your notes for one day might look something like this:

Observation	My thoughts	How I found out more and what I found out	Further action	What I have learned
Today I noticed that people talk a lot about the weather.	Perhaps people talk about the weather because it is so cold here.	My mentor explained that people in Britain often open a conversation with a comment about the weather—it is a way of starting a conversation.	Today, I spoke with a patient. I told her that I thought the weather was cold. She said yes that it is cold for the time of year. I could see that it is normal to talk about the weather with British people. She seemed comfortable with this.	British people often start conversations with a comment about the weather—it is a good way to start talking to somebody.
Today I answered the telephone. The caller wanted to speak to one of the other nurses. I was not sure what to do, as personal calls were not encouraged in my country.	Things are different here, but I'm not sure what the rules are about personal telephone calls.	Again, I asked my mentor. She told me that it depends on how busy the ward is, but you can take a message too, if the nurse is busy. She also mentioned that nurses should not take too many personal calls, as this would stop important calls concerning patients coming through.	Today, I answered the phone. Again, the caller wanted to speak to one of the nurses. I asked who was speaking and went to find the nurse. She said that she was busy and could I take a message.	The rules about taking personal calls on the ward are not strict, but work-related calls are more important. The situation may be different on other wards or departments. I will make sure that I know what the policy is, if I work elsewhere.

As time goes on, you might find it useful to start collating your findings under headings, such as:

Use of English in informal situations ('chatting')

Use of English in more formal situations

Working with others

Clinical procedures

Ways of behaving

As stated on Page 14, you could expect your cultural map to continually change as you add to it.

Activity 2

A Reflective Exercise

The purpose of this activity is to reflect on different interactions, to identify any areas of misunderstanding and to learn from them, including the best ways of dealing with them.

The people you talk to will depend on your individual situation: where you are working or studying or both. The following is an example, and could be adapted accordingly:

Who I spoke to today	What I was happy about	Any misunderstandings on my part	Any misunderstandings on their part	Action	What I have learned
A patient					
A relative					
A nurse					
A doctor					
A healthcare assistant					

Here is what part of your reflective activity might look like:

Who I spoke to today	What I was happy about	Any misunderstandings on my part	Any misunderstandings on their part	Action	What I have learned
A doctor	The doctor asked me about a patient and I was able to give him the information he needed.	I did not understand what he asked me first of all—he had an accent that was difficult to understand. I had to ask him to repeat the question. I felt a bit nervous asking him this but he did not seem to mind. He used a phrase that I did not understand— he told the patient that he wanted to 'run some tests'.	The doctor seemed to understand me.	1. I talked to my mentor about this situation. In my culture doctors are highly respected and this made me feel nervous about questioning him. 2. I re-read the chapter on 'communication and assertiveness.' 3. I am learning more about regional accents by watching the television. 4. I asked my mentor what 'run some tests' means and also consulted the chapter about idiomatic language.	1. It is OK to ask questions. 2. It is possible to be respectful and assertive at the same time. 3. I will become more used to regional accents as time goes on. 4. 'Running some tests' means carrying out clinical investigations.

Activity 3

Developing strategies for adaptation

Below is a list of possible strategies that could help you to adapt more comfortably to a new culture. These are based on the findings reported in the section above entitled 'Culture Shock'. Obviously, there will be individual differences in the way that people cope with change; some people will find some suggested strategies helpful while others will find the same strategies unhelpful. This activity is about identifying those strategies that you are most likely to benefit from.

List of strategies

- Rewarding myself (for example buying myself a new book or my favourite food) when I have had a hard day, or when I feel I have achieved something
- Seeking support from others in the same situation as me
- Trying to think positively
- Seeking support from somebody in a professional capacity, such a mentor or a tutor
- Making more effort to listen to others
- Making more effort to make new friends
- Keeping regular contact with friends and family in my home country
- Telling others more about how I feel
- Keeping occupied
- Going out more, for example sightseeing in my local area

- Going shopping more; this can include 'window-shopping' (this means just looking at what is available, not necessarily spending more money!)
- Finding out where I can practise my faith
- Visiting my local library to find out more about the local area and the country generally
- Seeking advice from people who have adapted well
- Looking for resources that may help me such as voluntary organisations.

Place these into columns as follows:

Those strategies that I have tried, and found helpful	Comments	Those strategies I have tried and did not find helpful	Comments	Those strategies I have not tried	Comments	One strategy that I will try this week	Comment

An extract from your activity might look something like this:

Those strategies that I have tried, and found helpful	Comments	Those strategies I have tried and did not find helpful	Comments	Those strategies I have not tried	Comments	One strategy that I will try this week	Comment
I went to the local town and spent an afternoon walking around the shops on my own.	I was surprised to find this activity enjoyable and useful. I was interested to see what differences there were between what is available here and at home. There were a lot of people around and I liked feeling part of a crowd. I was able to practise talking to people.	Making more effort to make new friends	I would like to do this, but find it difficult to talk to people to the extent of making friends with them. Most of the people I know are from my country. I think I need to learn more about ways that people begin conversations. I intend to explore ways of socialising more.	Visiting my local library	I think this may be useful, but I need to find out where the library is, and how to get there. Perhaps people at work will know, or I could look it up on the Internet.	Making more effort to listen to others	I think this links in with making new friends. On my course we have learned that it is important to develop listening skills, and that people feel valued when you listen to them.

This is an activity that you could build on as time goes on, by constantly reflecting on and evaluating your progress. For example, if you decided to adopt the strategy of making more effort to listen to people as in the example above, after a week you could look back and consider whether or not this has been effective.

Chapter 2

Idioms, colloquialisms, euphemisms and regional variations in the use of English

Communication difficulties can arise when students from overseas encounter idiomatic and colloquial language.

An **idiom** is a word or phrase which has a meaning that is commonly understood between a group of people, but which may have a different meaning from its original. An example is 'she is feeling under the weather' which means that she is not feeling very well. An Adaptation student from China reported that she read in a newspaper the phrase 'chalk and cheese', and did not know what it meant. This phrase is used sometimes to emphasise the difference between two people, as in: 'The husband and wife are as different as chalk and cheese'.

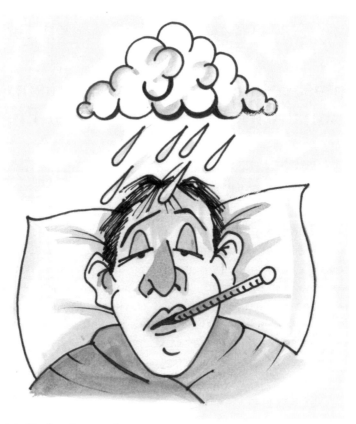

Figure 2.1: Under the weather

A **colloquialism** is a word or phrase that is informal, a version of 'slang'. It may, in some cases, be derogatory or offensive. An example of a colloquialism is: 'He has a dickey heart', which means that he has a heart problem. There is a special kind of colloquial language, called Cockney Rhyming Slang. This originated in the East End of London, but the odd phrase has spread to a wider usage. An example is 'Mince Pies', which means 'eyes'. Sometimes the rhyming element is omitted, which makes the slang even more mysterious. An example is: 'whistle'. This is short for 'whistle and flute', which is cockney rhyming slang for 'suit'.

A **euphemism** is known as a 'figure of speech'—using one word or phrase to replace another, often in the interests of avoiding the use of an unpleasant word or phrase, such as referring to 'the toilets' as 'the ladies'. Another euphemism was identified in *Chapter 1* applying more specifically to practice as 'not for the team', meaning that an individual is not for resuscitation. The purpose of this could be to conceal the unpalatable meaning of this label from patients.

Idioms, colloquialisms and euphemisms do not usually translate literally, and are often meaningless to somebody whose first language is not English.

It may be helpful to think of some examples of idioms and colloquialisms in your first language (if English is not your first language). This may help you to get used to the idea of idiomatic and colloquial language.

Within the healthcare profession, you are more likely to encounter idiomatic language, rather than colloquial language. However, you may well encounter colloquialisms among some patients, or even relatives.

You will learn more about idiomatic and colloquial language as time goes by, during the course of your working and social life.

Other unfamiliar words and phrases

Some words and phrases, which sound unfamiliar to you, do not fit neatly into the categories of idiom, colloquialism or euphemism. I was talking to a group of Adaptation nurses from India about the management of conflict. When discussing a scenario, I mentioned that I had adopted 'a bottom-up approach'. The group began to laugh, as they had never heard this phrase before. In this context, 'a bottom-up approach' means facilitating staff to resolve a conflict by getting them to identify issues and develop problem-solving strategies between them, rather than using 'a

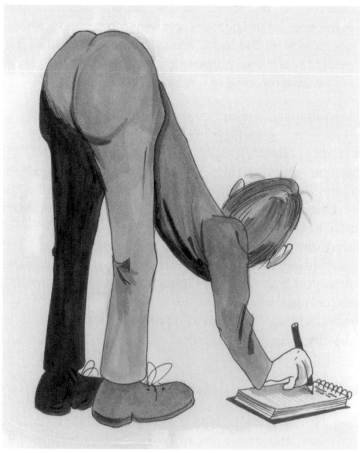

Figure 2.2: A bottom-up approach?

top-down approach' which would be more prescriptive and authoritarian.

Our language evolves constantly. Each time a dictionary is updated, new words and expressions are added. These often reflect our contemporary way of living. The latest Concise Oxford English Dictionary contains 900 new words. One new expression that is health-related is 'health tourism'. This means travelling to improve one's health, for example by visiting a health spa, or travelling to another country for healthcare, perhaps to obtain treatment more quickly, or more cheaply.

Regional variations

As with other countries there are regional variations in the use of English throughout the United Kingdom. **Dialect** refers to the use of vocabulary by a specific group of people. There is increasing mobility within the UK, and as a result we are more exposed to different regional variations in relation to the use of English.

Shifts in the use of spoken English have led to changing attitudes towards Received Pronunciation (RP). RP has previously been thought of as the type of English that an educated upper-middle- to upper-class person would speak; the Queen speaks in this way—that is why it is sometimes referred to as the 'Queen's English'. Previously, only people who spoke this way would be employed as television and radio presenters. Nowadays, the media has played a powerful role in promoting the acceptance of regional variations in English language, by enabling people with regional accents to become more accepted as television and radio presenters.

The relevance of all this for you is that you will be able to listen to a variety of accents via the media, which you may find helpful in terms of being introduced to different regional variations.

Summary

- Communication difficulties may arise for international healthcare students when they encounter idiomatic, colloquial or euphemistic language that they are unfamiliar with.

- Idioms, colloquialisms and euphemisms all involve a different use of words and phrases from their original meaning.

- You are more likely to encounter the use of idioms and euphemisms within the workplace. Colloquialisms tend to be less formal and can sometimes be offensive.

- You may encounter some other unfamiliar words and phrases as our language evolves constantly. You may find it helpful to use an up-to-date dictionary.

- There are regional variations in the way that people speak. Presenters with regional accents within the media have become more acceptable and it is therefore possible for you to learn more about regional accents by watching the television and listening to the radio.

Activities

Activity 1

Quiz

Select the idiom that is most likely to be used in place of the word or phrase in brackets:

1. When we arrived at the scene of the car accident the driver was (near death):

   (a) taking a turn for the worse (b) back on his feet (c) at death's door (d) going under the knife

2. After walking home in the rain I (became sick with) a cold:

   (a) broke out in (b) came down with (c) took a turn for the worse with (d) blacked out with

3. My father is (healthy again) after his recent illness:

   (a) back on his feet (b) under the weather (c) breathing his last (d) at death's door

4. Although the man was very sick I think that he will (recover):

   (a) run a temperature (b) throw up (c) pull through (d) take a turn for the worse

5. After eating the seafood at the restaurant, the man began to (vomit):

   (a) throw up (b) pull through (c) breathe his last (d) break out

Answers can be found on page 121.

Activity 2

Look for examples of idioms, colloquialisms and euphemisms in some newspapers. Ask somebody to explain them to you. You might also find it helpful to look them up on the Internet. In some instances, you might get a result just by typing the phrase into the 'Google' search engine. You could also try:

http://www.peevish.co.uk/slang/

Activity 3

Make a note of any words or phrases that you hear, but don't understand both at work and outside of work. Use the same strategy as for Activity 2 to find out what they mean.

Chapter 3

Communication and assertiveness

Some students from overseas have reported that they find it difficult to be assertive.

A group of Adaptation nurses from India reported that they are not accustomed to challenging authority. When faced with criticism, they would tend to question their own ability rather than consider challenging the person who has delivered the criticism, even if that criticism might not be justified.

There could be cultural differences in the way that different modes of behaviours are interpreted. For example, within one culture, it may be considered quite normal to converse loudly. To outsiders, this could be interpreted as two people engaged in an argument, displaying aggressive behaviour.

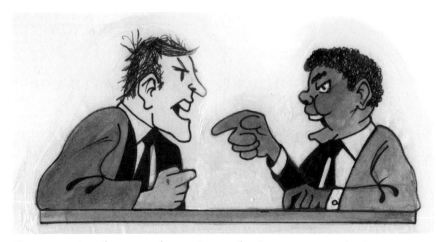

Figure 3.1: Are these people arguing, or having a conversation?

Assertiveness is considered alongside three other modes of behaviour, which are less effective. This helps us to make comparisons, and to become aware of behaviour that can help us to be more effective in both professional and personal interactions. The other three modes of behaviour are:

- Being aggressive
- Being passive
- Being manipulative.

We shall briefly consider these, before looking at assertive behaviour in more detail.

Being aggressive

Being aggressive includes some or all of the following behaviours:

- Shouting
- Using inappropriate language
- Insulting somebody
- Using physical force
- Not listening to the other person
- Being intimidating.

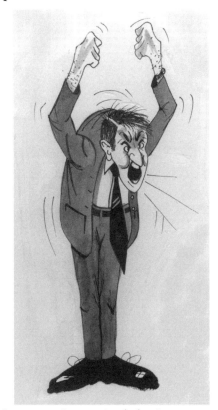

Figure 3.2: Aggressive behaviour

Being passive

Being passive includes some or all of the following behaviours:

- Being afraid to say 'no'
- Being afraid to challenge somebody
- Being afraid to ask for what one wants
- Being submissive.

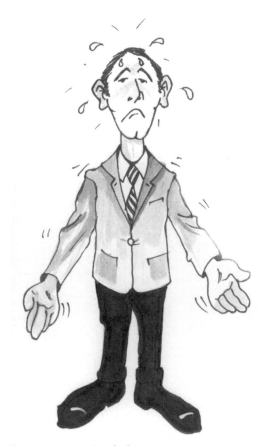

Figure 3.3: Passive behaviour

Being manipulative

Being manipulative includes some or all of the following behaviours:

- Playing on the weaknesses of others
- Being dishonest
- Being insincere
- Being flirtatious
- Giving false promises
- Using bribes.

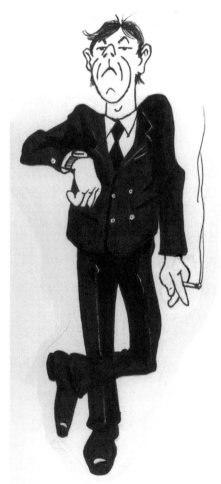

Figure 3.4: Manipulative behaviour

Each of these three types of behaviour is inappropriate for different reasons. Aggressive people may get what they want up to a point, but many of us do not want to respond to this type of behaviour. If a person adopts an aggressive mode of behaviour, they may lose control of a situation, which is a key factor in being effective. There is also an ethical aspect, in that aggressive behaviour involves demonstrating a lack of respect to others.

Passive behaviour is likely to be the least effective. Passive people can become vulnerable as others learn to take advantage of them.

As with aggressive behaviour, there is an ethical dimension to be considered in the use of manipulative behaviour. It involves dishonesty, which again may be effective up to a point, but this can be short-lived once others become aware that this type of behaviour is being used.

The most effective behaviour is to be assertive. Key features of assertive behaviour are:

- Being honest
- Being straightforward
- Being direct
- Being precise
- Not being afraid to say 'no'
- Respecting the views of others
- Taking responsibility for one's beliefs and actions.

Some students comment that they believe that they have used all four types of behaviour. This could be true, although we tend towards one type or another. The assertion that we are capable of using all modes of behaviour suggests that we have the capacity to develop our assertiveness skills.

As a student of healthcare, you are likely to encounter a variety of different situations and people throughout your educational programme. If you are unfortunate enough to encounter a situation wherein you feel that you have been treated unfairly by somebody, you should feel able to challenge them. Many students report that they feel uncomfortable about doing this. Some say that if they challenge somebody, for example a mentor, then their assessment or report will be affected. Ironically, this is often not the case because the person challenged (should the reason be genuine) becomes aware that they need to modify their behaviour.

Case Study

Student X approached her personal tutor because she was concerned about the way that the ward manager on her current placement was treating her. She felt that he was finding fault with her unnecessarily, and she did not like the way he spoke to her in front of other staff. She did not want the situation to continue, but also did not feel confident to challenge him.

The student's tutor helped the student to devise a strategy to address this problem, using a structured approach.

- The tutor pointed out to the student that if no action was taken, then the situation would be likely to continue. The ward manager is likely to have treated others in the same way, and if this is the case, would continue to do so. The manager is in effect being given permission to carry on being a bully. Bullying and harassment take a variety of forms, and are increasingly being recognised as issues that sometimes need to be addressed within the workplace. However, the tutor was careful to respect the views and fears of the student and took time to discuss these with her, stressing that she would support the student whether she decided to challenge the ward manager or not

- Using the principles of assertive behaviour, the tutor advised the student not to respond in kind to the ward manager, for example not to shout back at him in public. She advised her to approach him and ask to speak to him in private, at a specific, mutually convenient time; to make an appointment with him

- In the event of the ward manager not cooperating with this request, the tutor advised the student to put her request for a meeting into the form of a letter. The written word can be quite powerful and may gain a result when the spoken word fails

- Should the ward manager still not agree to a meeting, then it would have been time for the student to mobilise other sources of support. She had already approached her personal tutor, who could then have acted to ensure that the situation did not continue, with a variety of possible scenarios; perhaps by liaising with the appropriate person to bring about a transfer for the student. The tutor would have been able to remind the student that a planned system of support is available—represented as a flow chart, jointly devised by both school and service representation

- In this scenario, the manager agreed to a meeting. The tutor advised the student to make a note of the issues she wished to discuss prior to the meeting. This helped her to remember all the points she wished to discuss, and to keep the meeting on track

- The tutor advised the student that, again in keeping with the principles of assertive behaviour, she should be very precise and specific about her grievances. It is not helpful to make generalised statements such as: 'You are always being horrible to me'. It is more effective to say 'I do not like the way that you criticise me in front of other staff'. This is also an 'I' statement, for which the student is taking responsibility

- The student should allow the ward manager an opportunity to speak and to present his side of the story. There may have been a misunderstanding, and there may possibly be some degree of justification for criticism (although not in relation to the way the criticism was delivered)

- The student should aim to agree some outcomes from the meeting with the manager; for example, they may agree that the manager would in future refrain from criticising her in front of other staff and that the student would work with her mentor to develop her skills in identified areas

- The student should then put the agreed outcomes in a politely worded letter to the ward manager, inviting him to respond in writing. As stated previously, the written word can be powerful and also acts as evidence in the event of the situation continuing

- If this strategy fails then, as described previously, the student should access other sources of support. Ideally, she should inform the ward manager of her intentions in this respect.

The outcome of this scenario was that the student reported back to her tutor that she had found the courage to approach the manager, and the situation had improved.

The principles of the above scenario can be adapted to a variety of different situations, related both to work and to life outside of work.

Summary

- There may be cultural differences in relation to our interpretation of behaviour. Our cultural background may also have influenced our beliefs about authority.

- Assertive behaviour is considered alongside aggressive, manipulative and passive behaviour. This helps us to understand effective behaviour by comparing it to behaviour that is unethical and/or less effective.

- Key features of assertive behaviour are being open, honest, straightforward, precise and respectful of the views of others.

- Within our everyday lives, both in work and outside of work, we encounter situations that require us to be assertive. Learning to be more assertive can increase our effectiveness in all aspects of our lives.

- Many of us find it difficult to challenge somebody. However, once the initial step has been taken, the outcome can be very effective.

- It is possible to adopt a structured approach towards confronting somebody in an assertive manner. It is important to stay in control and to be clear about what you want to happen.

Activity

Carry out a Critical Incident Analysis

To do this you need to think of an incident involving an interaction with another person, which you think was successful for you, or one that you were not happy about. Either way, these incidents can be valuable learning opportunities. Here are some examples:

- You tried to tell a healthcare assistant on the ward that you did not agree with her moving and handling technique, but she was not very responsive
- You spoke to a relative about a complaint he made and he responded very positively
- You tried to complain about poor service in a restaurant, but you were unhappy about the outcome
- You returned some goods to a shop and successfully obtained a refund, after some initial reluctance on the part of the staff.

It is best to choose an incident that has a definable beginning and end. You should then write down what happened. Using the following framework, you can then analyse the incident:

- Do you consider that your action was appropriate?
- If not why not?
- How do you feel about what happened?
- What did you learn from the incident?
- What would you do differently next time?

This framework has been adapted from the work of Burnard and Morrison (1994).

Doing this makes you look at your behaviour more objectively, so that you can learn what is effective and what is not. Notice that the framework asks you to think about the way that an incident made you feel. Emotions are very important—strong emotion can have an effect upon the way that you deal with a situation, and can affect rational thinking.

Chapter 4

Study skills, part I

Two chapters have been devoted to the subject of study skills. This chapter examines some basic skills which can be developed, based upon the principles of English for Specific Purposes education (ESP) which was introduced in the Introduction, Page xvii. Some activities are provided, using a text-based approach. These are intended to increase your awareness of different ways of writing and to provide you with some practice in written English.

The next chapter considers some more specific issues in relation to writing academic essays and examination technique.

According to Hutchinson and Waters (1996), ESP is an approach to language teaching in which all decisions as to content and method are based on the learners' reasons for learning, hence the 'specific purposes'.

International healthcare students have very specific needs in relation to communication and cultural adaptation. Their priorities are likely to be:

- Adapting to a different culture, in the wider sense (see Page xviii)

- Adapting to the more specific culture of healthcare within the wider cultural context (see Page xviii)

- Gaining specific communication skills

- Coping with the demands of being a healthcare student in terms of meeting the requirements of the theoretical and practical components of their educational programme.

These priorities are interlinked in some ways. This chapter will focus mainly on the study skills aspects—the last bullet point—but in doing so will also address the other points, which have been covered elsewhere within this book.

Case Studies

The following three case studies illustrate different ways in which cultural issues can impact upon the individual's ability to study.

Aisha is from Somalia and has lived in the UK for about five years. She is studying by distance learning for a module which is part of a pathway leading to a degree in Health and Social Care. English is not her first language.

Aisha found that her studies have been quite culturally biased, in that examples used to illustrate various points were based on what she describes as an 'English culture'. Some historical examples have been used within her course, which seem strange to her, because she originates from a different culture.

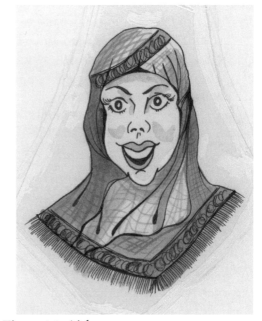

Figure 4.1: Aisha

There is growing awareness that we need to consider the cultural context within which we develop learning materials and lesson plans. In the meantime, you could make a note of any examples used within lectures, teaching materials, books or journals that you do not understand and discuss these with your teacher or personal tutor.

Nantale is from Uganda and has lived in the UK for about 18 months. She is a qualified nurse and is currently attending a Continuing Professional Development research module in order to improve her research knowledge and skills.

Nantale considers that her cultural background affects her ability to write an essay. This is because she tends to write in what she calls a 'direct translation format'. She feels that in her culture people speak in a circuitous manner. Because this mode of speaking is what she is accustomed to, she tends to write essays in this way also. She feels that the marker may then be distracted from the point of the essay by her inability to write concisely and succinctly. These qualities are often valued as part of essay-writing. This is reflected by the fact that essay guidelines usually stipulate a word-limit (see Activity 3, page 58).

Magdalena is Spanish. She is currently undertaking a module by distance learning that can be used towards a degree in Health and Social Care. Although she has lived in England for ten years, she still experiences some communication difficulties. She says that her 'biggest concern is that I cannot stick to the word allowance'. This is a similar issue to the one highlighted by Nantale. She says this is because she feels she needs to explain her ideas properly in order for anyone to understand her point. Again, Activity 3 on page 58 provides an opportunity to practise skills in writing concisely.

Text-based teaching

Text-based teaching grew from the Systemic-Functional Grammar model of language (Knight, 2001). The rationale for text-based teaching is that language occurs as whole texts, which are embedded in the social contexts in which they are used; in this case, the context is healthcare.

As stated in the Introduction (page xvii), ESP teaching is used with mostly adult students who already possess a level of what is described as 'language control'. Rather than focus on detailed issues, such as grammar and spelling, language in the form of whole texts (which can be spoken or written) is used to familiarise the student with certain ways of speaking and writing within a different culture.

There are different methods of analysing texts. Firstly, we can consider the context within which a text has been constructed, in terms of situation and culture. This is represented by Figure 4.2.

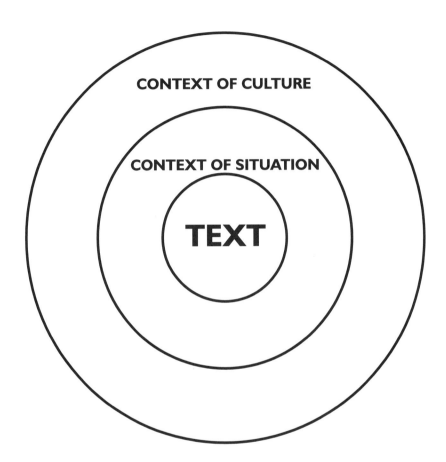

Figure 4.2: Text in context (Butt *et al*, 2000)

The uniqueness of a piece of language arises from the combination of its context of situation and context of culture. To illustrate this, I will use the example of 'giving a lecture'. I have lectured in different environments, in five different countries, at various levels. The 'context of situation' could be a college, a university or a clinical area, among others. 'Situation' could also refer to aspects of the environment, such as the type of classroom; for example, a small seminar room, or a large lecture theatre. 'Cultural context' could refer to the geographical setting, but could also refer to culture in a microscopic sense (see page 3), such as the prevailing 'culture' of a particular university, which may embrace certain values, which in turn influence approaches to education.

Imagine that I am to give a lecture on communication skills. The 'text' will be constructed according to the contexts of situation and of culture, and could be quite different within different contexts.

Aisha (Page 46) referred to educational materials that were culturally contextualised and were therefore unfamiliar to her.

We can understand more about the situational contexts of texts by considering what are known as the 'parameters of context of situation'. These are called field, tenor and mode. These can be explained by using the example of an essay written by a healthcare student:

Field: What the text aims to achieve (to meet assessment requirements)

Tenor: The relationship between writer and reader (which could also, in some incidences, be between speaker and listener) (student and marker)

Mode: The type of text created (an essay)

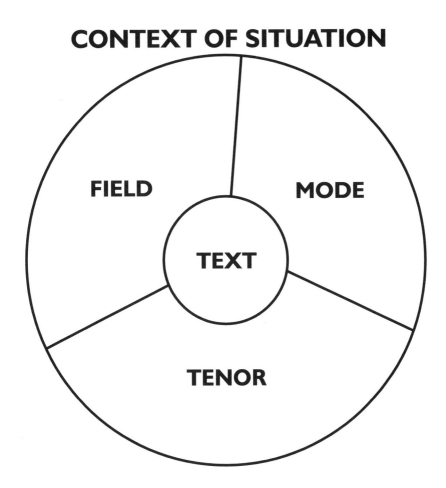

Figure 4.3: Parameters of context of situation (Butt *et al*, 2000)

Only one of these parameters has to change for the text to become something quite different. Let us imagine you have produced such a good essay that your teacher suggests you could submit it to a healthcare journal for publication. It is unlikely that it will be acceptable in the format that was appropriate for assessment purposes; it would probably need to be adapted to suit the 'house style' of the journal in question—the length of the text may need to be changed, for example.

We can now see that texts are constructed in different ways according to the purpose for which they are intended. The main purpose of this chapter is for you to be able to recognise and hopefully construct an appropriate text-type for essay-writing purposes.

Using the principles of systemic functional linguistics, texts can be placed into one of seven categories (Burns *et al*, 2001). The results of a study conducted by the author revealed that the text-types most commonly used within a sample of British health-related literature were:

Discussion

Exposition

Procedure

Discussion

This involves looking at an issue from different perspectives before reaching an informed conclusion. Many if not most written essays should be based on this text-type.

Exposition

This differs from discussion, as the starting point is what is known as a 'statement of position'—there is only one perspective. An example could be an aspect of the law, for example, relating to the storage and administration of drugs. It is important that healthcare practitioners are aware of such issues in the interests of patient safety and the consequences for themselves of failing to adhere to policies and procedures. Exposition could in some cases be an appropriate text-type to use within an essay, depending on the subject matter.

Procedure

This involves telling the reader or listener how to do something. In healthcare, there are many clinical procedures, which will vary according to the individual's speciality or discipline but could include:

- Recording a blood pressure reading
- Testing a urine sample
- Changing a wound dressing
- Recording a radial pulse
- Bathing a patient
- Administering medication.

Procedures are central to the healthcare practitioner's role, whatever their area of interest. There are many books and journal articles devoted to clinical procedures. Research leads to changes in practice as our knowledge grows, for example regarding what we know about the most effective hand-washing techniques. Technology has also had an impact upon some clinical procedures, for example with the introduction of electronic and digital blood pressure recording devices.

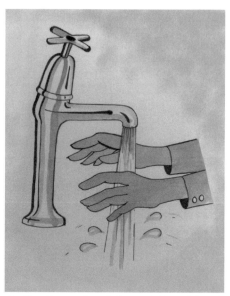

Figure 4.4: This is indicative only of the activity of hand-washing and does not necessariloy represent accurate technique

What do we know about the most effective hand-washing techniques? The author's research identified that some procedures have been written in a way that might not be clear to all; this could include international healthcare students. Some texts were ambiguous and lacked detail, which could be confusing or quite simply insufficient in terms of information-giving. Some texts are better than others. It is worth looking out for those that include rationales (explanations or reasons) for each stage of a procedure that is identified. This helps the reader to understand the purpose of each stage of a procedure (the 'why' behind the 'what' and 'how'—see page 70). It is also a good approach to use when writing an essay that involves procedures. I have found the *Fundamentals of Nursing* text by Taylor *et al* (2005) to be helpful in this respect.

Ideally, procedures should be taught and learned in a 'mixed mode' fashion. This means that you should learn a procedure by a series of processes that could include:

- Theoretical input
- Demonstration
- Practice in a 'safe environment', such as a clinical skills laboratory
- Practice under supervision within a clinical setting.

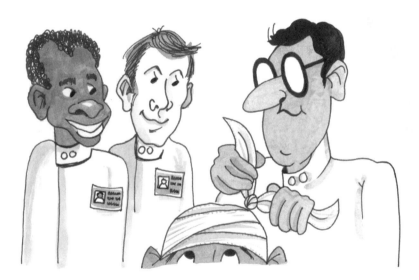

Figure 4.5: Demonstration

The above stages should be complemented by the student's own reading. As mentioned previously, procedures are often updated so it is necessary to keep up to date with any changes. Some procedures can only be performed by qualified practitioners, and so new skills are developed after the individual has gained his or her basic qualification.

Local procedure guides should always be consulted and adhered to as these may vary.

We will now focus on applying the discussion text-type to essay construction. The discussion text-type has three basic structural elements:

- The issue under discussion

- Arguments for

- Arguments against.

The following is an extract from a textbook about clinical procedures (Mallett and Dougherty, 2000) on the subject of using hot air dryers after hand washing.

Structural elements	Text
Issue	The use of hot air dryers
Arguments for	One study found that electric air dryers were very effective in removing Escherichia Coli and rotaviruses from washed hands (Ansari *et al*, 1991)
Arguments against	Hot air dryers which dry hands slowly and in some cases, inadequately (Matthews and Newman, 1987) may discourage some people from washing their hands (Blackmore, 1987). However, electric hand dryers can disperse bacteria for about 1m around the dryer, which suggests that dryers are unsuitable for use in critical patient care areas (Ngeow *et al*, 1989). This view is supported by Gould (1994a).

Figure 5.5: The use of hot air dryers (Mallet and Dougherty, 2000)

You can see that there is one argument in favour of the use of hot air dryers, and two arguments against, although one of these pertains to a particular clinical area. Although this is a very brief extract, it gives a clear example of presenting arguments for and against an issue, and is indicative of what the informed conclusion is likely to be, that hot air dryers are contra-indicated.

Furthermore, the arguments used are *evidence-based*; that is, the authors of relevant research papers have been cited. The argument against, relating to the dispersal of bacteria, is further strengthened by reference to more than one relevant study.

This short extract provides a very good model for the way in which essays should be written. You should demonstrate evidence of argument and analysis and your discussion should be supported with relevant reference to the literature.

Summary

- English for Specific Purposes (ESP) approaches aim to develop communicative competence for students who have specific needs, for example international healthcare students who need to develop communication skills in relation to the culture and practice of healthcare, as well as the wider cultural context.

- A segment of language is referred to by functional linguists as a 'text'. A text is constructed within both situational and cultural contexts. Texts are constructed according to the purpose for which they are intended.

- ESP adopts a text-based approach to enable students to make sense of language as whole texts that exist within a cultural context.

- There are different text-types. Within a sample of literature, three test-types were found: discussion, exposition and procedure. Procedures are central to the role of the healthcare practitioner, but the discussion type reflects the need for healthcare practitioners to be reflective and analytical. The exposition text-type is used when there is less room for debate, such as with issues relating to the law.

- The discussion text-type provides a good model for essay writing. The student should present different perspectives, which should be evidence-based.

Activities

Activity 1

Pick an article at random from a journal that you have used in your capacity as a healthcare student. Try to analyse it in terms of its parameters of context of situation, field, tenor and mode (see Pages 49–51).

Activity 2

Look through some journals that you have used in your capacity as a healthcare student. An example could be the *Nursing Times*. Try to identify articles that have been written using the discussion text-type. For each article, identify the issue, the arguments for and arguments against. Identify whether or not the arguments have been supported with reference to relevant research findings.

Activity 3

Write 300 words entitled 'On being an international healthcare student in the UK'. Try to adopt a discussion style. You can include your own experiences as well as those of others, by making reference to the literature, but try linking these together. Structure the essay to include a brief introduction and conclusion. Aim to include four references. If possible, ask a mentor or tutor to read the essay and comment on it. On page 121, there is a 'model answer' to give you some ideas if you find this activity challenging. However, your essay could be very different from the model answer and still be acceptable.

Some students find it difficult to write concisely, which clearly you will need to do to write a meaningful essay using only 300 words. Nantale (Page 47) spoke about her tendency to speak and write in a circuitous manner. Part of this exercise is to try to write exactly 300 words. One way of doing this, assuming that you write more, is to go through the essay and try to find ways in which you can take words out or rewrite parts of the essay more concisely. The model answer gives one example of how this was done.

Chapter 5

Study skills part II: essay writing, distance learning and examination technique

Assessment requirements will vary, according to the programme, course or module that you are following, and specific guidelines will be provided by the programme, course or module leader.

However, many healthcare programmes, courses or modules require students to write essays. There follow some general principles for essay writing, which the author has developed as a result of marking hundreds (if not thousands!) of essays with a range of healthcare programmes at different levels. The principles are headed as follows:

- Guidelines

- Terminology

- Individuality

- Structure

- Confidentiality

- Giving reasons

- Referencing.

Later, some examination techniques will be discussed. Many of the principles of essay writing apply also to answering examination questions (those that are required to be in essay format).

Some thoughts are also offered on the particular challenges of studying via distance learning.

Guidelines

The essay should be written according to the guidelines/criteria provided. Some programmes will provide more detailed guidance than others. The Open University, for example, offers very structured guidance to students following a second-level healthcare module, as part of an undergraduate degree programme. In some programmes, the percentage weighting is provided for each requirement. For example, some pre-registration nursing programmes specify the expected content, broken down into components of an essay, together with the highest number of marks out of 100 that could be awarded for each component. For example, let us imagine that you have been asked to write an essay about the care of a patient or client over 24 hours. One of the marking criteria could be:

Discuss the role of the nurse 30%

This means that roughly a third of your essay should be devoted to discussing the role of the nurse in the care of the patient over 24 hours. In the interests of equity, both the marker and the student are provided with the criteria and percentage weighting. For this reason, these may be collectively referred to as a marking guide.

Terminology

The example marking criterion above includes the word 'discuss'. This word gives you an indication about the style that should be adopted when writing this section of your essay. This also applies to examinations. The last chapter specifically addressed the discussion style of writing (pages 56–57).

Other words you may encounter in essay or examination questions might include:

- Identify
- List
- Compare
- Explain
- Critically analyse

The terminology used will vary according to the level of the programme that you are following. For example, the ability to 'critically analyse' is quite an advanced skill, which you would develop as you follow higher-level programmes of study. To critically analyse means that you can combine original thought and theoretical input (the published work of others—see *Referencing*, page 70) to consider a particular topic from various perspectives, in some depth. At the other end of the scale, to 'list' means just that—to provide an appropriate list of items that are asked for. For example, you could be asked to list the signs and symptoms of a myocardial infarction (heart attack), which could include:

- Moderate to severe chest pain
- Dizziness
- Shortness of breath
- Nausea
- Radiating pains in the arms and chest.

Individuality

We aim to help healthcare students to view patients and clients as 'whole' people. That is, they are people with physical, psychological, social, emotional and spiritual needs. This means that we have moved away from task-orientation (which would involve nurses and other healthcare workers, for example, approaching patient care as a series of physical tasks to be carried out; i.e. taking temperatures or bed-making) towards patient-centred care, which involves the nurse or health worker viewing the patient or client as a whole person with a range of needs to be met. This has resulted in key worker and named nurse systems being developed, which involve nurses and other carers looking after the total needs of a smaller group of patients, rather than focusing on the physical tasks associated with a larger group of patients or carers. Previously, the patient was primarily viewed in terms of their condition; 'the broken leg in bed 8'. This rather simplistically reduced patients to what was physically wrong with them, and stripped them of their individuality. Caring for people as complex beings with a range of needs is reflected in the way that assessments are now structured. For example, instead of having 'myocardial infarction' (heart attack) as the central focus of an essay question, the patient would be the most important consideration. The patient may have had a myocardial infarction, for which he or she must be treated, but there are other considerations that could have an impact upon their condition, such as psychosocial factors. When writing an essay, therefore, it may be helpful to write it with the patient or client uppermost in your mind. In doing so, you are respecting their individuality.

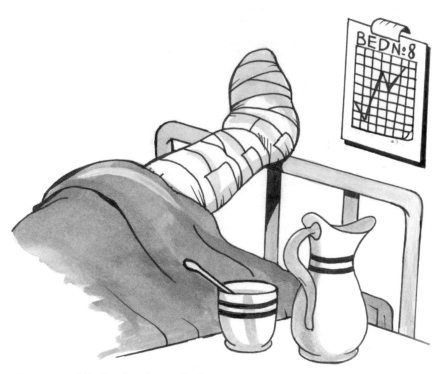

Figure 6.1: 'The broken leg in bed 8'

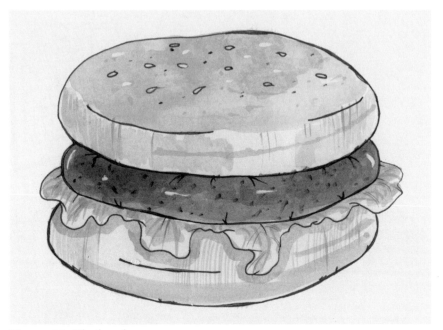

Figure 6.2: The hamburger

Structure

The essay should be structured in that it should have a clearly identifiable introduction, main body and conclusion. One teacher described this structure as a 'hamburger'—the meat represents the main body which needs to be held together above and below by the bread roll, which in turn represents the introduction and conclusion. Without the bread roll, the hamburger falls apart. Without an introduction and conclusion, the essay is also incomplete.

The introduction

In order to clearly demonstrate to the marker that you have included an introduction, you could begin with something like:

'The purpose of this essay is to...'

or

'This essay will include...'

The introduction can be used to set out your intentions in terms of the content and development of the essay. It could help to demonstrate how you intend to 'manage' the essay. Essay guidelines usually include a word limit, which you should keep to, to within ten per cent. For example if the word limit is 2000 words, your word count should be somewhere between 1800–2200 words. This does not usually include the reference list, or any appendices.

Some students struggle with a word limit; they find it difficult to say what they want to say, within the constraints of a set number of words. They find it difficult to be concise. The introduction can, therefore, be used to convey to the marker the way that you intend to approach the essay, but in doing so you must ensure that this approach has covered all of the marking criteria. (See Activity 3 on page 58, Chapter 4 for practice writing concisely.)

Here is an example of an introduction to the essay about the care of a patient over 24 hours:

The purpose of this essay is to discuss the care of a 74-year-old male patient, named Harry (name changed to protect the confidentiality of the patient), over a time period of 24 hours following admission to the ward. Harry has been admitted to the ward with a diagnosis of myocardial infarction. The background of the patient will be described, and its relevance to his care and treatment. The possible causes, signs and symptoms of myocardial infarction will be identified as this forms the basis of health education for Harry, as well as our understanding of the condition. The assessment of Harry will be discussed, using a nursing model as a framework, and his care described, having assessed his needs. The role of the multiprofessional team will be identified. The central theme of this essay relates to the safety and comfort of Harry. The use of a nursing model will emphasise the need to consider Harry's needs holistically...

Conclusion

The conclusion can usually be quite brief, but expressed in a way to demonstrate that the essay does not just end abruptly. The conclusion should summarise the most important points and draw together the key arguments. As with the introduction, you could begin the conclusion with something like:

'To summarise...'

or

'In conclusion...'

This should draw the marker's attention to the fact that you have included a conclusion.

Here is an example of a possible conclusion to the essay about Harry:

To summarise, the priorities for Harry were identified as follows: to monitor his condition and to prevent his condition from becoming worse; to protect his pressure areas because of his age and because he was immobilised; to establish a treatment plan; to educate him about his condition; and to reassure both him and his wife, who was very anxious. The first 24 hours of care are critical in all these respects. In order to address these priorities, it was essential that the multiprofessional team was involved in Harry's care and early rehabilitation process.

Confidentiality

In the example of an introduction (page 67), confidentiality was referred to. When writing an essay, you may be asked to write about a patient or client you have worked with. This may be referred to as a 'case study'. You must protect the identity of the patient. This applies also to the identities of relatives or staff. Not only must you protect their identity, but you must also make it clear to the marker that you have done so. A pseudonym was given to Harry. This protects his identity but at the same time helps us to view him as a person.

Giving reasons

In the example introduction on page 67, you should notice that some rationales are included. This means that you go one step beyond making a statement, to giving a reason for the statement. You should aim to do this within your essays. An example from the sample introduction is:

The possible causes, signs and symptoms of myocardial infarction will be identified as this forms the basis of health education for Harry.

If the student had limited this sentence to its first part, then this would have been informative up to a point, but not educational—it would have stated the 'what' without including the 'why'.

A useful summary of a basic approach towards writing an essay is to continually ask the following, in this order:

- What?
- How?
- Why?

In relation to the essay about Harry, you would identify what your action will be, how you will carry out the identified action and why you are carrying it out. Remembering these three words, in this order, could prove a useful tool when writing essays and exam answers.

Referencing

If your chosen healthcare programme includes essay writing within its assessment strategy, then you should receive information about how to reference your work. Some students do seem to experience difficulties with referencing, so some general points will be addressed here.

Why reference?

Referencing involves giving evidence that you have done some reading of published books or journals around a particular subject. Sometimes unpublished work is used, such as degree dissertations. It is necessary to acknowledge the source of any information that you have obtained from a published or unpublished source, otherwise you could possibly be penalised for plagiarism.

Plagiarism essentially means the copying of material which is then presented as the writer's own work. The original source is not acknowledged. Some students plagiarise unintentionally, because they are unaware of the regulations. Some markers will overlook initial incidents as early mistakes, and will advise the student to take care in the future. Essentially, plagiarism is a form of cheating, and must be avoided.

How to reference

There are two acknowledged referencing methods: Vancouver and Harvard. You should be advised which one to use, together with instructions about how to use them. The method refers to the way that work is referenced both within your essay, and also within the reference list at the end of your work. A reference list refers to the citations you have made within your essay. A bibliography refers to any background reading you may have done that is not directly cited within your essay.

Distance learning

For those of you who are studying via distance learning, there are some particular points which can help you to complete your course successfully. I have studied in this way and am also a tutor for a distance learning module, and it has become clear that this mode of learning presents certain challenges (although it also has many advantages, in relation to accessibility and flexibility), for example:

- Because of the nature of distance learning, you are bombarded with a huge amount of paperwork (unless the course is an online programme). It is quite easy to miss important pieces of information. Try and organise your paperwork; for example, use a filing system or a system of folders for different aspects. Be quite ruthless in discarding anything that you think you can do without (but be a 100 per cent certain that it is not important!).

- Mark down deadlines in a place where you will see them—you may not have any other reminders.

- Try to attend tutorials, if applicable. This can be motivating because you get to meet other students, who are in the same situation as you are. You may receive useful input for assessments and exams. Attendance can be helpful in giving you the impetus to see the course through—it becomes something that is more 'real'—distance learning can seem an almost abstract concept that is difficult to comprehend.

- Maintain contact with other students (more likely if you attend tutorials)—students often gain comfort and encouragement from each other, as peers.

- Seek alternative methods of support if unable to attend tutorials, for example through the Internet. Maintain contact with your tutor—this may be via email. If you ever feel low, or about to give up, that is the time to contact your tutor (or perhaps other students as well).

- Try not to get behind with work: extensions are possible, but students who do not keep up are probably those who are the most likely not to complete.

- The organisation you are studying with may offer support for students with special needs (in fact they are particularly good in this area), and for students for whom English is not their first language. This support is worth accessing. The Open University is very good in this respect.

- Ultimately, despite any amount of support, the responsibility for completing the requirements of the course lies with **YOU**, the student. This can be quite an isolating realisation; stick with it, and if necessary be assertive if you feel that you are not receiving the right amount of support in any area.

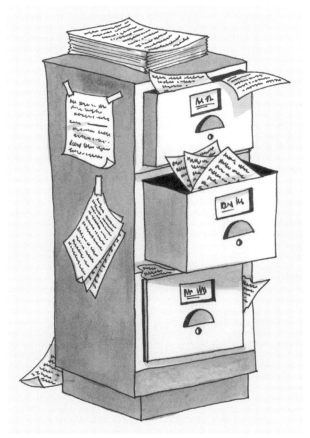

Figure 6.3: Organise your paperwork

Examination technique

Not all readers will need to sit an examination; this section is intended only for those of you who will be taking written exams, for example pre-registration student nurses. Nobody ever believes me but I think that sitting an examination can be almost an enjoyable experience. My best experience of sitting a written exam was when I felt prepared. I actually enjoyed answering the questions and felt a sense of satisfaction at the end.

This section will cover the following aspects of examination technique:

- Preparation
  - practical issues
  - revision
  - brainstorming with peers
- The actual exam
  - timing
  - planning
  - interpreting the question
  - constructing your answer.

Preparation

Practical issues

Part of the 'de-stressing' strategy is to get the practical issues out of the way. There are things that you can do well in advance and others, nearer the day.

Well ahead be sure that you know the **date, time** and **venue** of the exam. Block out your diary. If the venue of the examination is new to you, research and plan the journey so that you will arrive in plenty of time. You could even consider a practice run.

Nearer the time, gather together what you will need for the exam; for example, pens, pencils, erasers and ruler, a form of identification if required.

As difficult as this may be, try to get a good night's sleep before the exam—being tired can significantly affect your ability to concentrate and to retrieve information. Again, from my experience, I feel that it is easier to sleep well if you feel confident that you are *prepared*.

The night before the examination, set out everything that you will need. This saves last minute panic the next day. You could even decide what you're going to wear so that your clothes are ready. The aim is to minimise any last-minute setbacks, such as not being able to find your keys.

Revision

Ideally this should start well ahead of the exam.

The starting point should be looking at past questions (specimen or past papers). Specimen or past papers might be provided for you by your programme leader or may be available in the library. You could then plan out model answers to these questions, using the technique of brainstorming (see below) or by devising mind maps (see page 82), both as an individual and as a group exercise. The purpose of using specimen or past papers for revision purposes is that, although your exam questions may not be exactly the same, there will be some repetition in relation to content. What might vary is the angle you are expected to take. The question itself gives clues in this respect—addressed on page 84.

Once you have model answers (expressed as bullet points rather than full essays), you can use these as the basis for your revision.

Brainstorming with peers

This is a way of preparing for examinations with other students. The potential benefits are that:

- Part of your preparation is done in cooperation with others which may help to reduce any sense of isolation—revision can be a lonely activity

- 'Two (or more) heads are better than one'—the group may generate more ideas than one person can.

You could meet up with some of your fellow students during your revision period.

Using past papers, the group brainstorms aspects that could be covered by simply contributing any ideas that come to mind. One person should write down all the ideas. The group then discusses what has been said and develops a model answer. I have used this technique in revision classes, and it has worked well.

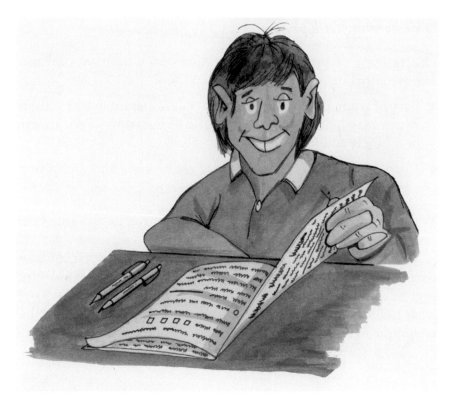

Figure 6.5: Exams can be fun!

The actual exam

Timing

Timing can be crucial to examination success. The following section details an approach to timing that requires a degree of self-discipline.

The length of the exam will vary according to the course that you are following, the type of exam, or the stage of the course (in that some courses have exams at the end of each year).

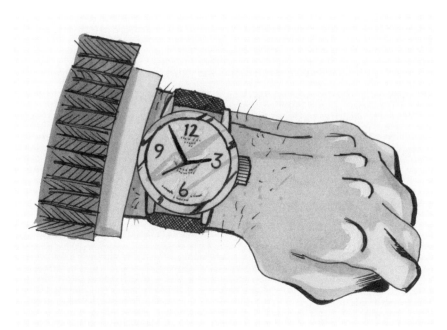

Figure 5.5: Timing is crucial

For the purposes of this suggested technique, it is assumed that the exam is three hours long, and that you are required to answer three questions. Adjustments can be made accordingly.

Rather than simply allowing one hour per question, time should be allocated for:

- Reading the instructions
- Selecting the questions you will answer (if given a choice)
- Planning your answers
- Checking your answers.

If you do not allow time for these activities, one of more of the following outcomes might happen:

- You might misunderstand the instructions (it has happened!)

- You might choose to answer a question that is not right for you. If you do this you might then decide to abandon it halfway through in favour of an alternative question. Valuable time will have been lost

- You might not construct your answers in a logical sequence

- You might not have time to notice and correct any mistakes

- Your work may appear untidy if you have not allowed time for planning, as you have to scribble last-minute thoughts in between existing lines.

You could allocate 50 minutes for the actual writing of an answer. This leaves a total of 30 minutes for reading the instructions, selecting the questions, planning each answer and checking each response. Obviously timing will need to be adjusted according to the actual length of the exam and the number of questions to be answered.

If you get to the end of your allotted time for an answer but have not finished, you should stop and move on to the next question. You can go back to the unfinished question later. This means that you pay equal attention to each question. I have marked papers which indicated that the student spent a lot more time on one question than another.

If you think that 30 minutes sounds like a lot of time to spend not actually writing the answer, then it may be worth thinking in terms of this time as an investment into the planning of the question. Once this groundwork has been done, the writing part should be a lot easier.

Planning

This leads on to the subject of planning an examination answer. When you are in an examination room, you may find it difficult to concentrate. Your instincts may tell you to just start writing, without planning. This could lead you to produce a response that lacks a logical progression and to omit relevant content.

It is a generally accepted practice to be able to write your plan onto the answer sheet, to head it as 'plan' and then put a line through it prior to handing in the paper, to indicate to the marker that it is not part of the final examination answer. You could discuss this with your tutor prior to the exam, or ask the invigilator on the day of the exam before it starts, to be certain that this practice is acceptable.

Two methods of planning for examination questions will be discussed here. The first involves brainstorming and the second method involves using a mind map. For this purpose the following question will be used:

The concepts of curing and prevention within healthcare are interrelated. Discuss this statement.

(This question has been invented for illustration purposes and has not been taken directly from any previous examination papers.)

Brainstorming

This is often a group activity, but as you are working alone in the examination room you can adapt the technique. Basically, you should write down any word or phrase that comes into your head that is associated with the main themes of the exam question. You should be guided by the keywords (see page 84). When you run out of ideas, go through your list and organise it into order of priority. This helps you to structure your essay. In relation to the question, brainstorming may generate the following ideas:

- Healthcare: what is it
- Curing: define
- Prevention: define
- Prevention of diseases
- Cure of diseases
- Examples of diseases, e.g. cancer
- New diseases: are they curable and/or preventable?
- Ethics of curing and preventing disease
- Technology
- Economics: which is more cost-effective—prevention or cure?
- Self-cure
- Individual responsibility for health
- Different types of prevention
- The role of the media in health prevention
- Media-information about curing.

Mind maps

According to the principles of Neuro-Linguistic Programming (NLP), we all have different ways of processing ideas; for example, some of us think in pictures, whereas others may think in more abstract ways (Andreas and Faulkner, 1996). This could influence our preferred method of planning. If you think graphically, then you may prefer to use mind mapping.

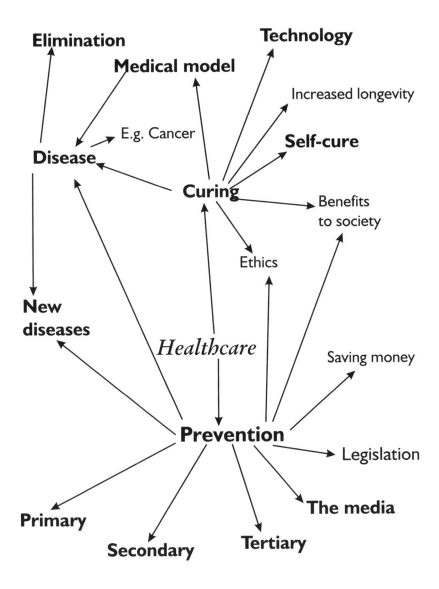

Figure 5.6: Mind map

Mind maps evolve from a central idea which branches off into topics from which ideas can be generated. Figure 5.6 is an example of a mind map that was generated from the sample question.

The central concept used for the mind map is 'healthcare'. This leads to the two themes of 'curing' and 'prevention'. These in turn lead to different ideas, some of which apply to both themes. This helps us to think about the ways in which curing and prevention may be interrelated; for example, there may be ethical and economic issues that apply to both.

Interpreting the question

The more you practise this, the less likely you will be to misinterpret the question in the exam room. Remember that feeling nervous may cause you 'not to see'. As stated previously, you are more likely to feel calm if you have prepared thoroughly for the exam.

Having selected your question, part of the question planning should be to identify the **keywords** in the question:

The concepts of <u>curing</u> and <u>prevention</u> within <u>healthcare</u> are <u>interrelated</u>. <u>Discuss</u> this statement.

Note that the word 'discuss' is also underlined. The reason is because this word indicates the style you should adopt when writing the answer. Other words which are indicative of style of writing are listed on page 63 of this chapter.

The remaining underlined words indicate that the following should be addressed:

- You should demonstrate an understanding of the concepts: 'curing' and 'prevention'

- You should discuss ways in which these concepts are interrelated

- Your discussion should be located within a healthcare context.

How your answer should be constructed

As with an essay, your exam answer should include an introduction and a conclusion. You should use the introduction to indicate how the answer will proceed. For the example question above, an introduction could be something like this:

> *Within this essay the concepts of curing and prevention will be explored. The ways in which these concepts may be interrelated will be considered. The discussion will be located within a healthcare context, using specific examples to illustrate the arguments made.*

In this introduction, deliberate use of the language found within the exam question has been made. The message to the marker is that you are speaking the same language and have picked up the 'clues' given in the question. This does not mean that the introduction repeats the question but rephrases it and adds another relevant dimension in the form of 'specific examples'.

Summary

- It is important to obtain information from the organisation you are studying with in relation to the specific assessment regulations that apply there. This includes the preferred referencing method.

- Both essay and examination questions contain 'clues' about the way in which the answer should be written, in the form of keywords.

- When writing about a patient or client, they should form the main focus for your answer; in doing so you are respecting their individuality. You should not disclose the identity of the patient. Any staff or relatives referred to should also remain anonymous.

- Essays and written exam answers should be structured with an introduction, a main body and a conclusion.

- Within essay and exam answers, reasons should be given throughout for actions or ideas expressed. The basic repetitive structure of What, How and Why should be applied throughout.

- It is essential to avoid plagiarising by acknowledging all sources of reference used within an essay.

- Studying via distance learning presents a particular set of challenges. You need to be quite self-disciplined but should seek support when necessary.

- The stress of examinations can be reduced by careful planning and preparation.

- It is helpful to study for exams with other students to reduce the feeling of isolation and to generate ideas.

- Careful timing and planning during an examination can optimise your chances of passing.

Activities

Here are some strategies to maximise your chances of producing essays that will gain you a pass mark:

- Keep in close contact with your personal tutor (if applicable) from an early stage of your course. Ask him/her to look at draft essays and to give you feedback. Every time you get an essay back look carefully at the comments made and try to make an obvious attempt to respond to them in the next essay. Markers often look favourably on assessments that indicate that the student has clearly responded to feedback. Marking systems will differ between courses. In some courses your allocated tutor will mark your papers; elsewhere papers will be marked by specialist tutors depending on the subject matter of the essay. There will always be a system of moderation and some external examination. The purpose of both is to ensure that students' work is marked fairly. If for any reason you cannot ask a tutor to look at your work, ask another teacher, a colleague or even a friend. It is important that somebody else can read your work and understand it. A 'critical reader' may also pick up errors associated with written expression of English.

- See if you can find some examples of essays previously written by other students that are of a good standard. Try the library or ask your tutor, or even other students. These will give you an idea of what you should aim for in terms of academic standard. A word of caution: do not use this opportunity to plagiarise, as that is a serious academic offence (see page 70)

Glossary

It is important to note that the meanings given for the terms within this glossary are specifically relevant to the context of this book—some of the terms used may have different meanings within other contexts.

Abbreviation

A word or phrase shortened often, but not always, by using initial letters. An example is TTAs referring to (prescribed) medications to take away (on discharge from hospital).

Accent

Pertains to those features of pronunciation which are indicative of an individual's origins.

Access programmes

Approved Access programmes prepare adult learners for admission to some courses that would otherwise require formal qualifications as entry criteria.

Adaptation nurses

Nurses from overseas who are already qualified but who need to undertake a period of supervised practice and an induction programme prior to becoming eligible to practice as a registered nurse within the UK.

Admissions interview

An interview conducted by a nurse with a patient following their admission to a clinical area, for the purpose of gaining information that will enable the patient to receive comprehensive care and treatment, and will also offer an opportunity for the patient to ask questions and to receive reassurance.

Aggressive behaviour

When compared with assertive behaviour, refers to behaviour that involves being intimidating and disrespectful.

Alienation

Feeling that you are separate from a situation; this may result from hostility shown towards you.

Ambiguity

Refers to an expression that has more than one possible meaning.

Analysis

Studying a subject by breaking it down into component parts.

Anonymity

Ensuring that individuals' names are not attached to information held about them. For example, when writing about patients within an essay, a pseudonym or initial should be used to protect their anonymity. This ensures confidentiality.

Appendix

Supplementary information that is placed at the back of a piece of work (for example, a written assignment) and is not included within the word count. The plural form of this word is appendices.

Argument

A point of view which may be for or against a particular topic. The argument within an essay should be evidence-based.

Assertive behaviour

A type of behaviour that involves asking for what you want in an effective way that remains respectful of others.

Assessment

Judging the ability of a student in a particular area using set criteria.

Assignment

A piece of work, for example an essay, that a student is expected to complete in order to meet the assessment requirements of a course of study.

Asynchronous (communication)

Refers to a type of communication which involves the receipt of a message being delayed and therefore the response to the message being delayed. An example could be leaving and accessing a voicemail message.

Avoidance

Making a conscious effort not to engage with people.

Beliefs

Ideas which reflect our view of the world; our individual interpretation of truths.

Bibliography

A list of books and journals located at the end of a piece of work (for example, an essay) that does not contain references that have been used within the text, but which have been used as background reading.

Brainstorming

A method of generating ideas. Individuals are allowed to contribute any associative thoughts that come into their head. This allows for creativity. The ideas generated can then be refined.

Bullying

An act of intimidation; an attempt to dominate, often directed towards a person who is more vulnerable.

Care plan

A written plan formulated by a healthcare professional after a patient has been assessed. The plan provides a detailed outline of the person's needs and the care required to meet those needs.

Case study

The meaning of case study can vary according to its context, but can be applied to the study of an individual patient in order to learn more about their condition, care and treatment. Within this book the term 'case study' has been used to describe the experiences of international healthcare students in order to identify issues and strategies.

Circuitous

A circuitous route is one that deviates from the most straightforward one. To speak or write in a circuitous manner is to express oneself in a roundabout way, not being straight to the point.

Client

A term that is used as an alternative to 'patient' in some settings which places emphasis on the individual as a person who is receiving a service.

Clinical procedures

Guidelines for a wide range of procedures used within healthcare, such as wound care and recording a blood pressure. Some clinical procedures can only be performed by qualified healthcare practitioners; some require additional training such as venepuncture (drawing blood with a needle from a vein).

Clinical setting

Any setting in which the care and treatment of patients take place, such as a hospital ward or an outpatients department.

Clinical skills laboratory

A facility which contains equipment, such as blood pressure devices and resuscitation models, which enables students to practise clinical skills in a safe environment prior to implementing them in supervised practice.

Cockney rhyming slang

A particular type of colloquial language which originated from the East End of London; for example 'Apples and pears', meaning 'stairs'.

Colloquialism

A word or phrase which may also be referred to as 'slang'. A type of informal speech. An example is 'hanging out' with your friends—meaning that you are spending time with them.

Communication

Shared meaning; the transmission and understanding of verbal and non-verbal information.

Communicative competence

A level of skill that requires not only linguistic ability but also the ability to understand the cultural framework of a language.

Concise

To be concise is to be brief and to the point while still being informative. To write concisely is to include as much information possible using the fewest words possible. This does not necessarily mean writing in note form; it may still be necessary to write in complete sentences, according to individual assessment requirements. The word 'succinct' has a similar meaning.

Confidentiality

Refers to access to information about an individual. For example, access to patient information is restricted to authorised personnel, which is required to enable them to be able to treat and care for the patient. For this reason, when patient information is used for the purpose of an essay, their identity must not be disclosed so as to prevent unauthorised people gaining access to information about them (ensuring anonymity).

Consent

Permission: can refer to a patient giving consent for an operation. Within this book, individuals have given consent for their experiences to be described (although their identities have been protected; see: anonymity and confidentiality). The issue of informed consent is important; individuals give consent once all the relevant information has been given to them, so that they understand the consequences of having given consent.

Continuing Professional Development (CPD)

An ongoing programme of learning that qualified practitioners undertake in order to remain updated within their profession. In nursing this is a mandatory requirement.

Contra-indicated

A particular drug may be contra-indicated for people who have certain conditions; in other words it is advised that the drug may not be suitable for some people.

Coping strategies

Behavioural and psychological techniques, that people adopt in order to reduce the effects of stressful situations.

Counsellor

This can have different meanings, but in this context refers to a person who is trained to listen to somebody's problems, maintaining confidentiality and to guide them towards problem-solving.

Criteria

A set of statements against which a judgement is made. For example, marking criteria guide both student and marker in relation to the expected content and standard of a written assignment. Criteria is a plural word; its singular form is 'criterion'.

Critical analysis

A skill which a student is expected to demonstrate when writing essays. This expectation applies to students studying at degree level or at a more advanced stage of their educational programme. For example, pre-registration student nurses are expected to develop this skill as their course progresses. Critical analysis involves adopting a questioning approach, and drawing upon theory to support arguments made and conclusions reached. The use of critical analysis within academic work is a skill that can be applied to practice, in terms of questioning practice and one's own performance.

Critical incident analysis

A tool for reflecting on professional practice that involves selecting an episode that 'stands out' for some reason, which may seem positive or negative, describing the incident and how it made you feel, then analysing and learning from the incident in order to improve on practice, or to become more effective in terms of personal development.

Critical reader

A person who takes an objective look at somebody's written work, for example an essay, prior to submission for marking. They may be asked to comment on one aspect, such as the use of English.

Culture

A concept that is not easy to define but which embodies the observable features of a society or an organisation, such as behaviour as well as those elements that are less visible, such as values and beliefs.

Cultural adaptation

A process that should follow on from culture shock when the individual uses coping strategies to adapt to a new culture, without losing sight of their own cultural identity.

Cultural bias

Similar to cultural specificity, but with a more negative connotation. Cultural bias could refer to a mixed-culture situation that addresses the needs of one culture over another. An educational programme could be culturally biased if it has been designed with a particular cultural context in mind.

Cultural context

For the purposes of this book, this term could usefully be defined as 'the cultural information that surrounds a communication episode'.

Cultural map

A representation of 'the way that things are done around here', for example within the workplace.

Culture shock

A feeling of disorientation associated with being exposed to an unfamiliar culture.

Cultural specificity

The characteristics of something which make it meaningful and accessible for the members of a specific culture. For example, a healthcare service may be developed that is culturally specific for a particular ethnic minority group, or a book written that is aimed at a specific group.

Customs

The traditional practices of a group passed down from generation to generation.

Detachment

The preservation of a status of not belonging, by resisting involvement.

Dialect

A form of speech used within a particular region.

Discipline

An area of knowledge.

Discussion

Looking at a topic from different angles, perhaps in terms of disadvantages and advantages.

Dissertation

A substantial piece of work which is usually research-based, that is submitted in order to gain a degree. It may be referred to as a 'thesis'.

Distance learning

A mode of learning that involves studying from home, maintaining contact with a tutor via letter, telephone, fax and/or email. Some distance learning courses are conducted 'online' via the Internet.

Diversity

Differences between people, relating to such factors as age, race, religion and gender.

Educational programme
A recognised course of study.

English for Specific Purposes (ESP)
An educational approach towards teaching adults who already possess a level of competence in relation to the use of the English language, which focuses on the specific use of language within a particular context, for example healthcare.

Equity
Fairness; to enable all concerned to have an equal chance.

Essay
A written composition that meets assessment criteria.

Ethics
A code of behaviour based on beliefs about what is right and wrong.

Ethnicity
The heritage of a particular group that relates to one or more of the following: race, culture, nationality, religion.

Euphemism
The substitution of one word or phrase for another; often done to avoid the use of an unpleasant expression. An example is to say that 'he is at rest' instead of saying 'he is dead'.

Evidence-based practice
The use of research and evidence to guide clinical decision-making.

Examination technique

Strategies that can be used both prior to and during a written examination to increase your chances of passing, or excelling.

Exposition

Differs from discussion in that the topic has only one dimension; there is no scope for discussion, as in aspects of the law.

Field

What a text aims to achieve, for example to inform.

Figure of speech

An expression used to create effect by substituting one word or phrase for another. A euphemism is a type of figure of speech, although the use of a euphemism is usually to avoid unpleasantness rather than to create effect. An example of a figure of speech is to say that you are 'starving', when in fact what you mean is that you are hungry. The use of the word 'starving' is more dramatic, hence it creates an effect.

Flowchart

A graphical representation of a process which indicates the logical and correct steps to follow; an example is a flowchart of the steps to follow within a procedure, such as a complaints procedure.

Fundamentals of nursing

The basic, important aspects of nursing practice which a qualified nurse should be competent in. Some of these can then be taken to a more advanced level. There are many textbooks that have been written on the subject of the fundamentals of nursing.

Guidelines

A set of instructions that guide behaviour, for example in relation to assessment requirements.

Hand-over

The giving of information between healthcare practitioners, often between shifts, in order that all relevant information about patients is communicated, to enable the recipients of the information to deliver care accurately.

Harassment

Behaviour which is similar to bullying, which may be persistent.

Harvard referencing method

A method of referencing that involves including the author's surname and date of publication within the text and the full references listed alphabetically at the end. Some educational institutions specify which type of referencing system should be used. The student should seek more details about this method if using it.

Healthcare assistant (HCA)

HCAs work in hospital and community settings under the supervision of qualified nurses. They can undertake NVQ qualifications in order to have more responsibility within their role. Some HCAs go on to become qualified nurses once they have completed a programme of study for which they have the prerequisite entry requirements.

Healthcare practitioner

Any recognised healthcare professional; a provider of healthcare.

Holistic care

An approach to care that considers the 'whole person' in relation to their physical, psychological, social, emotional and spiritual needs.

House style

The requirements set by the publisher of a journal in relation to aspects of presentation in order to ensure consistency.

Idiom

A word or phrase which has a different meaning from its original, but is nevertheless understood by a group of people. An example is: somebody feeling 'under the weather', meaning that they do not feel very well.

Individuality

The recognition of identity by respecting the diversity of people in relation to such characteristics as gender, race or age.

Integration

Becoming incorporated into a community.

International healthcare student

Within the context of this book, an individual who has come from any country outside of the UK to study and/or to practise within the healthcare field.

Invigilator

A person who supervises students during an examination to ensure that they adhere to examination regulations.

Keyword

A word that is significant. For example, keywords within an examination question are those which give the student the best indication about the way that they should answer the question in terms of content and style.

Key worker

A healthcare worker who is assigned to work with a patient or client for a period of time, for example the duration of the patient's stay in hospital. A key worker could be a healthcare assistant (HCA).

Language control

A student who already has a level of (for example) English-speaking competence uses this to further develop their communicative competence by taking control of their learning and using the language in a confident way. Although this implies an independent approach to learning, a student can still be helped by others to reach this stage.

Lesson plan

The structured design of a lesson.

Macroscopic

Viewing something on a larger scale (for example culture).

Manipulative behaviour

Refers to a type of behaviour whereby an individual attempts to reach their goals by being dishonest and insincere.

Mentor

An individual who is usually more qualified and experienced who guides and advises someone less qualified and experienced. Mentoring relationships may be formal or informal.

Microscopic

Viewing something on a smaller scale (for example culture).

Mind map

A graphical representation of thought processes that allows ideas to be generated.

Mobilise

To put into action, for example to put a written policy into action.

Mode

The type of text created, for example a letter.

Model answer

A good example of an appropriate response to a set question, for example an examination question. There may be several possible responses that would meet the assessment requirements; a model answer is an example of the type of response that would result in a pass mark.

Moderation

A system of ensuring that assessments are consistent and fair.

Module

An academic unit of study. Modules vary in terms of the level of academic credit they carry and their academic level (for example diploma or degree level). Some modules are 'stand alone', that is they are recognisable as qualifications in their own right, but can also be used towards another qualification, such as a degree.

Multiprofessional team

Composed of different healthcare professionals, for example doctors, nurses and physiotherapists, who work together in relation to the care and treatment of the patient. Some teams include social care professionals also.

Myocardial infarction

Permanent damage to heart muscle caused by lack of blood supply to the heart, which may be referred to by lay people as a 'heart attack'.

Named nurse

A registered nurse who is responsible for the co-ordination of a patient's care.

National Vocational Qualification (NVQ)

The central feature of NVQs is the National Occupational Standards (NOS) on which they are based. NOS are statements of performance standards which describe what competent people in a particular occupation are expected to be able to do.

Neuro-linguistic programming

The study of human performance and excellence for the purpose of identifying skills which can be learned in order to improve effectiveness.

Non-verbal communication

Information expressed without the use of words, for example via gesture or eye contact.

Nursing model

A theoretical framework for nursing practice.

Open University (The)

An organisation established in 1971 that specialises in providing distance learning courses at different levels and in many different subjects, and which enables a wide variety of people to study in a flexible way.

Parameters of context of situation

Different aspects of a text relating to its aims, the relationship between the writer and reader (or speaker and listener) and its type.

Passive behaviour

A mode of behaviour which is characterised by timidity and submissiveness.

Pathway

In this book this term has been used to describe a series of modules which an individual can study towards gaining a degree qualification. The modules can be thought of as 'stepping stones' along the pathway towards gaining a degree.

Patient-centred care

An individual approach to patient care which includes working in partnership with the patient.

Peers

People who have something in common, who are equal in some way; often used in relation to age group or occupation.

Percentage weighting

A value assigned to a question, or a part of a question in an examination or other form of assessment. The value will be less than one hundred if the question is divided into sections with the overall highest possible score being 100. For example, 30 per cent may be assigned to a section asking the student to 'Discuss the role of the nurse...' as part of an overall question about the care of a patient.

Perspective

A way of looking at something; a view.

Philosophy (of care)

An accepted belief system associated with a particular discipline; in this instance, healthcare.

Placement (clinical)

A clinical area such a ward or an outpatients department to which a healthcare student is allocated in order to gain practical experience, while under supervision.

Plagiarism

Using the work of another author, for example within an essay, without acknowledging its source. Plagiarism is a serious academic offence.

Practice

Skills repeatedly used within a profession which are informed by theory.

Pre-registration student nurse

An individual undertaking a programme of study which will enable them to become registered nurses with the Nursing and Midwifery Council, if they have met the theoretical and practice requirements of the programme.

Prevention (health)

The term 'health prevention' tends to apply to public health activities such as immunisation and screening programmes. It may also be used in relation to the prevention of ill-health in more general terms.

Procedure

A set sequence of steps whose purpose is achievement of a goal. For example, a written clinical procedure such as recording a blood pressure is broken down into a series of stages for the purpose of recording a blood pressure result safely and accurately.

Programme leader

The person who manages an educational programme.

Pseudonym

An alternative name used to conceal the identity of a person.

Psychosocial

Pertains to social and psychological aspects of human functioning.

Rationale

An explanation; a reason; a justification. For example, when writing an essay, a rationale should be provided for each point that is made.

Received pronunciation (RP)
The regionally-neutral accent of British English which has traditionally been associated with the higher classes and private education. It is sometimes referred to as the 'Queen's English'.

Reference
The acknowledgement of a published or unpublished source of information cited within an essay. This is indicated both within the script and at the end of the essay.

Reference list
A list of all references that have been used within a text such as an essay, located at the back of a piece of work.

Reflective practice
Thinking about and critically analysing one's actions with the goal of improving one's professional practice.

Relaxation techniques
Methods intended to combat the effects of stress, such as the use of breathing exercises and relaxation tapes.

Revision
The process of reviewing coursework in preparation for an examination.

Safe environment
An environment such as a classroom which enables students to practise a range of skills prior to implementing them in supervised practice. The safe environment also enables students to discuss subjects in confidence.

Scenario

The descriptive and analytical use of a discrete situation which can be real or fictitious used to explain or illustrate a concept or topic. It may be used as a teaching aid. It is sometimes used with the future tense as in: 'there could be several possible scenarios...'

Second level module

Equivalent to the second year of a first academic degree (BA or BSc).

Situational context

The context within which a section of language (text) has been constructed; for example, the language used within a lecture depends on various situational aspects, such as the number of students and the type of teaching environment.

Slang

Informal language that is not standard. It may be abusive or coarse. It is also referred to as colloquial language.

Social care

There is some overlap between health and social care. Social care aims to meet the needs of vulnerable groups of people, ensuring that they have access to benefits and services to which they are entitled.

Socialisation

This word has two meanings that are relevant to this book. One pertains to meeting others for social purposes. The other meaning refers to adopting the normative behaviour patterns of a culture. A socialisation process occurs as a child grows up and learns behaviour from parents and significant others.

Study skills

Skills which include: planning a study schedule, taking notes effectively in class, revising for examinations, organising course materials and notes, examination techniques and essay writing.

Succinct

To write in a succinct manner is to explain something briefly. Has a similar meaning to 'concise'.

Supervision

Overseeing the work of another person who is usually less experienced and less knowledgeable.

Symbolic

Pertaining to the use of things which are observable; for example, items and pictures to represent concepts that are more abstract, such as belief systems.

Synchronous (communication)

Refers to a type of communication which is carried out with all parties present at the same time, but not necessarily in the same physical location, for example a telephone conversation.

Systemic-functional linguistics (SFL)

SFL is a social theory of language that looks at language in context at different levels of detail.

Task orientation

An approach to care as a series of tasks to be completed, for example bed-making or taking temperatures, as opposed to a patient-orientated approach which prioritises individual care.

Technology

In its broadest sense, technology refers to the 'practical application of knowledge', but we often think of the word in relation to technical tools, such as computers and mobile phones.

Tender loving care (TLC)

A phrase which is used to describe a special type of care which is often applied to terminally-ill patients. It prioritises pain relief and physical and emotional comfort rather than curative approaches to care.

Tenor

The nature of the relationship between the writer and reader, or between the speaker and listener, of a text, for example teacher and student.

Terminology

The words or phrases that are used within a particular discipline.

Text

A section of language which can be spoken or written.

Text-based approach

An approach to language teaching that considers language as whole texts which are embedded within a cultural context. The student learns firstly to recognise different types of text then progresses to constructing their own texts. This is an approach used within English for Specific Purposes (ESP) teaching.

Theory

Principles which inform practice.

Traditions

The practices of a group which have been in place for a long period of time.

Transmission

The act of sending a message.

Undergraduate

A student working towards his/her first academic degree.

'Underground' (The)

A train system based in and around London, large sections of which run underground. It is also referred to as the 'Tube'.

Values

Our ideas about what is good, and what is bad.

Vancouver referencing method

A method of referencing that involves the references within the text being represented numerically and the references at the end being listed numerically rather than alphabetically. Some educational institutions specify the use of a particular referencing method. The student should seek more details about this method if using it.

Voicemail

A voicemail system enables a caller to leave a verbal message if you are unable to answer the phone.

Vulnerability

An increased likelihood of being susceptible to exploitation or harm. Some groups of patients are considered to be more vulnerable than others, for example older people.

Word allowance

May also be referred to as a 'word limit'. This pertains to the minimum and/or maximum number of words you should use within a written assignment/essay, which is usually included within a marking guide or assessment guidelines. Rules vary between different guidelines so it is essential to be clear of individual requirements in terms of word allowance.

Resources

Websites

BBC World Service.com

- http://www.bbc.co.uk/worldservice/learningenglish/ index.shtml

Comments:

This is an excellent resource in terms of general English language support and cultural adaptation. It provides explanations of the vocabulary used within news reports, tips on pronunciation with sound, vocabulary and grammar, as well as links with other relevant sites. Highly recommended.

English Learner Newsletter

- http://www.angelfire.com/on/topfen/newsletter66.html

Comments:

This is a weekly email newsletter that is quite 'fun'. It includes quizzes, idioms and jokes, as well as useful links.

Skills for study

- http://www.palgrave.com/skills4study/html/non-english/ non-e_lectures.htm

Comments:

This is another good resource, which offers strategies to overseas students for getting the most out of lectures.

Using English.com

- http://www.usingenglish.com/speaking-out/ taking-control.html

Comments:

This is quite a resourceful site, which answers various questions in relation to the control of the English language and directs visitors to other useful sites, including some with audio links.

Books

Arakelian C, Bartram M and Magnall A (2003) *Hospital English: The brilliant learning workbook for international nurses.* Radcliffe Medical Press. ISBN: 1857758641

Comments:

This book is aimed primarily at Adaptation nurses, but all healthcare students should gain something from it. It is a very lively book with lots of activities, written by experts within the field of communicative competence in healthcare. It is very relevant as it addresses communication and culture issues within the healthcare context. Highly recommended.

Brink-Budgen R (2000) *Critical Thinking for Students: Learn the Skills of Critical Assessment and Effective Argument*, 3rd Edition. How To Books. ISBN: 1857036344

Comments:

This book should be suitable for many international healthcare students in terms of level of study. Chapters 4 and 5 highlighted the need for students to demonstrate evidence of analysis and argument within their essays. This book should be a useful resource in relation to helping students to develop these skills.

Murphy R (2002) *Essential Grammar in Use* with Answers and CD Rom. Cambridge University Press, Cambridge. ISBN: 0521529328

Comments:

This book has been recommended by a linguist who specialises in supporting students with developing effective written English. The CDRom contains 320 interactive grammar questions.

Reinders H and Lewis M (2003) *Study Skills for Speakers of English as a Second Language.* Palgrave Macmillan. ISBN: 1403900264

Comments:

This is an up-to-date book aimed at students at higher education level. The book is clearly written and very informative.

Salimbene S (1982) *Strengthening your study skills: A guide for overseas students*. University of London Institute of Education, London: ISBN: 085473144X

Comments:

This book is quite old but may be of help as it is specifically aimed at overseas students.

References and bibliography

Andreas S, Faulkner C (1996) *NLP: The new technology of achievement*. Nicholas Brealey Publishing, London

Arakelian C, Bartram M, Magnall A (2003) *Hospital English: The brilliant learning workbook for international nurses*. Radcliffe Medical Press, Oxford

Burnard P, Morrison P (1994) *Nursing Research in Action*. Macmillan, London

Burns A, Coffin C, Hall DR, Hewings A, Mercer N (2001) E841: Teaching English to Speakers of Other Languages. *Worldwide Study Guide*: 42; 128–31

Butt D, Fahey R, Feez S, Spinks, S, Yallop C (2000) *Using Functional Grammar: An Explorer's Guide*. Macquarie, Sydney: 9–13

Dudley-Evans T (1998) *Developments in English for Specific Purposes: A Multi-Disciplinary Approach*. Cambridge University Press, Cambridge

Gatehouse K (2001) Key issues in English for specific purposes (ESP) curriculum development. *Internet TESL J* **VII** (10):

Hortas J D (2003) *Choosing a Degree or English programme—English for Specific Purposes*: http://www.studyusa.com/articles/esp.htm; accessed: 5th July 2003

Hutchinson T, Waters A (1996). *English for Specific Purposes: A Learning-Centred Approach*. Cambridge University Press, Cambridge

Knight P (2001) The development of EFL methodology. In: Candlin, CN, Mercer N, eds. *English Language Teaching in its Social Context*. Routledge, London: 147–66

Mallet J, Dougherty L (2000) *The Royal Marsden NHS Trust: Manual of Clinical Nursing Procedures*, 5th edn. Blackwell Science, Oxford

Nursing and Midwifery Council (2002) *NMC Circular 30-2002—Standards for Supervised Practice*

Schon D (1983) *The Reflective Practitioner: How Professionals Think in Action*. Basic Books, New York

Soanes C, Stephenson A (2004) *Concise Oxford English Dictionary*, Eleventh Edition. Oxford University Press, Oxford

Taylor C, Lillis C, Lemone C (2005) *Fundamentals of Nursing: The Art and Science of Nursing Care*, 5th edn. Lippincott, Williams and Wilkins, Philadelphia

Answers

Answer

Chapter 3, page 31

Activity 1

Quiz on idioms
1. (c)
2. (b)
3. (a)
4. (c)
5. (a)

Model Answer

Chapter 4, page 58

Activity 3

On being an international healthcare student in the UK

The purpose of this essay is to explore some advantages and disadvantages of being an international student in the UK, using my own experiences and the findings of others to support the discussion.

I came to the UK three years ago to become a qualified nurse. At first I experienced difficulty in making myself understood, and understanding others. This is similar to the experience of Padilla-Harris (2001) who reported that she found it difficult to understand people who spoke quickly or who had regional accents when she first came to the UK.

It became clear to me that in order to understand people, I also needed to know more about their culture, as identified in the work of Briguglio (2000). Before I started my training, I worked for a while as a voluntary worker. This enabled me to meet many people and to adapt more easily to a different culture.

Leifer (2000) found that there are some negative attitudes shown by people in the UK towards healthcare workers from overseas. I have experienced some racism which upset me at first. However, when I started my training I met many other people in the same situation. We also learned about cultural issues and skills such as being assertive to help us to speak up for ourselves in an appropriate way. Witchell (2002) identified that some nurses from overseas might find it difficult to be assertive and may need help to develop assertiveness skills.

In conclusion, the advantages and disadvantages I have discussed relate mainly to cultural and communication issues. On the whole, I view coming to the UK to become a qualified nurse as a positive experience, because of a combination of my own determination and the support that is available to me, for example from my mentor and my tutor.

300 words (not including references, which are not usually included in a word count)

References

Brigulio C (2000) Generic skills: Attending to the communication skills needs of international students; Paper presented at the

10th Learning and Teaching Forum: Focusing on the student: Edith Cowan University

Leifer D (2002) Plain speaking. *Nurs Stand* **17**: 15

Padilla-Harris C (2001) Night fever. *Nurs Stand* **16**(5): 23

Witchell L (2002) Managing international recruits: managing an adaptation programme for overseas registered nurses. *Nurs Man* **9**(3): 10–14

Index